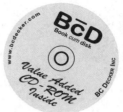
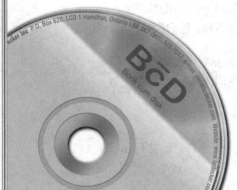

*PDQ** SERIES

---

*PDQ (Pretty Darned Quick)

PDQ PHARMACOLOGY

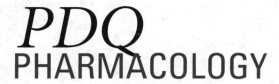

GORDON E. JOHNSON, PhD
Professor Emeritus

Department of Pharmacology
University of Saskatchewan
Saskatoon, Saskatchewan

SECOND EDITION

2002
BC Decker Inc
Hamilton • London

BC Decker Inc
20 Hughson Street South
P.O. Box 620, L.C.D. 1
Hamilton, Ontario L8N 3K7
Tel: 905-522-7017; 1-800-568-7281
Fax: 905-522-7839; 1-888-311-4987
e-mail: info@bcdecker.com
website: www.bcdecker.com

Previous edition copyright 1988.

02 03 04 / PC / 9 8 7 6 5 4 3 2 1

ISBN 1-55009-109-3

Printed in Canada

Sales and Distribution

United States
BC Decker Inc
P.O. Box 785
Lewiston, NY 14092-0785
Tel: 905-522-7017; 1-800-568-7281
Fax: 905-522-7839; 1-888-311-4987
e-mail: info@bcdecker.com
website: www.bcdecker.com

Canada
BC Decker Inc
20 Hughson Street South
P.O. Box 620, L.C.D. 1
Hamilton, Ontario L8N 3K7
Tel: 905-522-7017; 1-800-568-7281
Fax: 905-522-7839; 1-888-311-4987
e-mail: info@bcdecker.com
website: www.bcdecker.com

Japan
Igaku-Shoin Ltd.
Foreign Publications Department
3-24-17 Hongo, Bunkyo-ku
Tokyo 113-8719, Japan
Tel: 81 3 3817 5680
Fax: 81 3 3815 6776
e-mail: fd@igaku-shoin.co.jp

U.K., Europe, Scandinavia, Middle East
Elsevier Science
Customer Service Department
Foots Cray High Street
Sidcup, Kent   DA14 5HP, UK
Tel: 44 (0) 208 308 5760
Fax: 44 (0) 181 308 5702
e-mail: cservice@harcourt_brace.com

*Singapore, Malaysia, Thailand,
Philippines, Indonesia, Vietnam, Pacific
Rim, Korea*
Elsevier Science Asia
583 Orchard Road
#09/01, Forum
Singapore 238884
Tel: 65-737-3593
Fax: 65-753-2145

Australia, New Zealand
Elsevier Science Australia
Customer Service Department
STM Division
Locked Bag 16
St. Peters, New South Wales, 2044
Australia
Tel: 61 02 9517-8999
Fax: 61 02 9517-2249
e-mail: stmp@harcourt.com.au
website: www.harcourt.com.au

Foreign Rights
John Scott & Company
International Publishers' Agency
P.O. Box 878
Kimberton, PA 19442
Tel: 610-827-1640
Fax: 610-827-1671
e-mail: jsco@voicenet.com

Writing the dedication for a book is never easy,
particularly for a married man with six children. You know that each
and everyone of them will be looking in this space to make sure that his or
her name is here. So, to maintain our happy home, and pay all my
political debts, I dedicate this book to:

Mary-Jane (wife, mother, and benevolent dictator)
Dorothy
Ian
Warren
Louise
Ted
and
Becky

However, the story does not end here, for I
must also dedicate this book to the cascade of grandchildren
who have tumbled into our lives. For it is to these 12 products of
biotechnology that I owe my greatest debt. Thus, to Christina, Angela,
Gillian, Megan, Kelsey, Sarah, Vanessa, Victoria, Renee, Graham
(finally a boy!), Trevor, and Ryan, I dedicate this text. Who knows
what drugs we may have by the time they are in a
position to write their own books.

Preface

Pharmacology can be a most difficult subject to master. There appears to be so much to learn. Students can not be blamed if, overcome with the detail of individual drugs, they miss the basic concepts underlying the use of an entire group of agents. We encourage students to view our subject from a distance first, thus allowing an understanding of the basic principles of drug therapy before they commit to memory the properties of one drug after another. This is much easier said than done. It is hard to stand back and view the whole lake, if you are just learning to swim and are being swamped by each new swell. This book is intended to help beleaguered students, in danger of becoming "phagocytosed" by facts, rise above the field of battle and take a global view of complex topics. Only then can they return to the detail that is so important in correct drug use.

PDQ Pharmacology, is a small book. It is not intended to stand on its own. Rather, it is meant to complement a good general pharmacology text. Several excellent texts have been cited in this book. By the same token, this book should not be used as a substitute for a good undergraduate course in pharmacology.

If *PDQ Pharmacology*, is not intended to replace a recognized text or substitute for a course in pharmacology, how then should it be used? First, it can provide a valuable learning aid during the time the course is being taught. Filled with figures and tables selected to illustrate important principles of drug action, it will assist students to grasp the concepts that underlie groups of drugs before they are asked to concentrate on the properties unique to each agent. *PDQ Pharmacology*, can also assist students in reviewing pharmacology. In those last frantic hours prior to an examination, when students wish to review the entire course or require a rapid answer to an individual problem, *PDQ Pharmacology*, will fill the current void.

Gordon E. Johnson, PhD
March, 2002

Contents

Part 1   Principles of Medical Pharmacology

Drug Absorption, Distribution, and Elimination

CHARACTERISTICS OF DRUG MOVEMENT ACROSS MEMBRANES

Drugs are Dissolved in Body Fluids

Most drugs are either weak acids or weak bases. When dissolved in body fluids, they exist in both the **ionized** and **nonionized** forms. *The ionized form* is usually water soluble, or lipid insoluble, and does not diffuse readily throughout the body. *The nonionized form* is usually less water soluble and more lipid soluble. It is more likely to diffuse across lipid membranes (Figure 1–1).

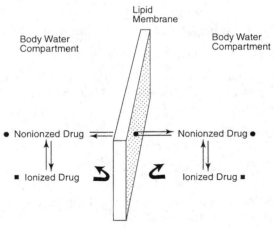

Figure 1–1 Diffusion of a drug across a lipid membrane. (After Johnson GE, Osis M, Hannah KJ. Pharmacology. In: Nursing Practice. Toronto (ON): W.B. Saunders, 1998.)

Ratio of C_i/C_n Drug Molecules

The ratio of ionized/nonionized (C_i/C_n) drug molecules depends on the pH of the environment and the pK_a of the drug in question.

Acids

$$HA \rightleftharpoons H^+ + A^-$$

$$C_n \qquad\qquad\qquad\qquad C_i$$

eg,   Salicylic Acid   Salicylate

When the pK_a of the drug = the pH of the media, then $C_i = C_n$.

Raising the pH has the effect of removing H^+ and driving the reaction to the right, therefore, increasing C_i. *Lowering the pH* has the effect of adding H^+ and driving the reaction to the left, therefore, increasing C_n.

Example: Salicylic acid has a pK_a of ~3.
At a pH of 3, $C_n = C_i$
At a pH < 3, $C_n > C_i$
At a pH > 3, $C_i > C_n$

Question: Would you expect salicylic acid to be mainly ionized or non-ionized in the stomach pH of 1?

Answer: Nonionized.

Bases

$$HB^+ \rightleftharpoons H^+ + B$$

$$C_i \qquad\qquad\qquad\qquad C_n$$

eg,   Morphine Sulfate   Morphine

When the pK_a of the drug = the pH of the media, then $C_i = C_n$.

Raising the pH has the effect of removing H^+ and driving the reaction to the right, therefore, increasing C_n. *Lowering the pH* has the effect of adding H^+ and driving the reaction to the left, therefore, increasing C_i.

Example: Morphine has a pK_a of ~ 8.
At a pH of 8, $C_n = C_i$
At a pH < 8, $C_i > C_n$
At a pH > 8, $C_n > C_i$

Question: Would you expect morphine to be mainly ionized or non-ionized in the stomach pH of 1?

Answer: Ionized.

OVERVIEW OF ABSORPTION, DISTRIBUTION, AND ELIMINATION OF DRUGS IN THE BODY (FIGURE 1–2)

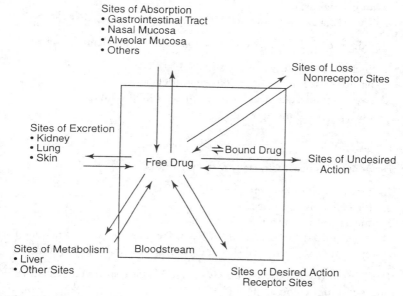

Figure 1–2 Characteristics of drug movement across membranes. (After Morgan JP. Alcohol and drug abuse, curriculum guide for pharmacology faculty. Rockville, MD: U.S. Department of Health and Human Services, 1985:3.)

ROUTES OF DRUG ADMINISTRATION

Sublingual

Drugs are absorbed through the oral mucosa. May be useful if a drug

1. irritates the stomach,
2. is destroyed in the stomach, or
3. is inactivated during its first pass through the liver.

Only an appropriate method of administration for a drug that

1. dissolves rapidly in saliva,
2. does not irritate the oral mucosa, and
3. is lipophilic.

Oral

1. Drugs are absorbed from the stomach and the duodenum.
2. Drug absorption is better from the duodenum because of its larger absorbing surface.
3. The stomach can absorb acidic drugs and weakly basic drugs.

For a drug to be absorbed from the stomach or the duodenum, it must

1. be dissolved in the gastrointestinal (GI) tract,
2. have at least 1 molecule in 500 nonionized, and
3. have nonionized molecules with sufficient lipid solubility to pass through the GI mucosa.

Rectal

Drugs are administered rectally for a systemic effect if

1. they are irritating to the stomach,
2. the patient is nauseated,
3. the patient is too young or old to take the drug orally, or
4. a sustained effect is desired (of less value today because of the development of sophisticated sustained-release oral and topical products).

Drugs are also administered rectally for a local effect, such as the treatment of proctitis or hemorrhoids.

Parenteral

Intravenous — immediate effect, danger of overdose.

Intramuscular — if the drug is dissolved in an aqueous media, absorption occurs rapidly; if the drug is administered as a suspension, absorption is prolonged.

Subcutaneous — absorption is almost as rapid as the intramuscular injection of a drug dissolved in an aqueous preparation.

Inhalation

For a systemic effect — effect starts immediately.

For a local effect — acts on the bronchioles.

DRUG DISTRIBUTION IN THE BODY

Initially

Drugs are carried in largest amounts to the most richly perfused tissues, such as the adrenals, brain, heart, lungs, kidneys, and muscles.

Later

Drugs then undergo redistribution within the body, being retained in tissues for which they have affinity, for example, in fat for lipophilic drugs (Figure 1–3).

Plasma Protein Albumin

Drug molecules may be bound to plasma proteins in the bloodstream, usually albumin. While bound to plasma proteins, drug molecules are inactive because they cannot leave the vascular system and enter the tissues. Once the level of free drug in the plasma falls, bound drug molecules diffuse off the plasma proteins in order to maintain a constant bound/free ratio (Figure 1–4).

Blood-Brain Barrier

Brain capillary endothelial cells have no pores to allow diffusion. In addition, glial connective tissue is attached to the basement membrane of cap-

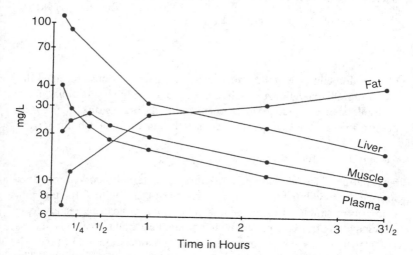

Figure 1–3 Time distribution of thiopental in a dog. Note the high levels found initially in the liver and the muscle, and the subsequent redistribution to fat. (After Brodie BB. Distribution and fate of drugs: therapeutic implications. In: Binns TB, ed. Absorption and distribution of drugs. Edinburgh: E and S Livingston, 1964:246.)

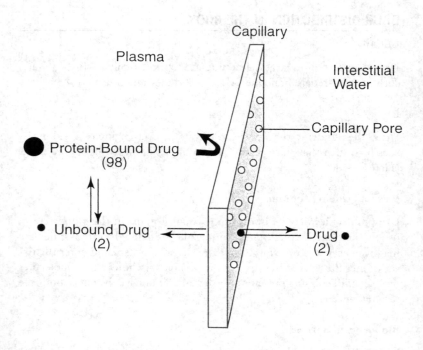

Figure 1–4 Schematic representation of the diffusion of a drug, which is 98% bound to plasma protein, across a capillary. (After Johnson GE, Osis M, Hannah KJ. Pharmacology. In: Nursing Practice. Toronto (ON): W.B. Saunders, 1998.)

illary endothelium. Together, these structural modifications are called the blood-brain barrier. Ionized molecules cannot enter the brain. Nonionized molecules, not bound to plasma proteins, enter the brain easily (Figure 1–5) because they are lipid soluble and can pass through the blood-brain barrier.

Placental Transfer Of Drugs

The mature placenta contains a network of maternal blood sinuses that interface with villi that carry the fetal capillaries. Drugs cross the placenta primarily by simple diffusion. Lipid-soluble, nonionized drugs readily enter the fetal blood from the maternal circulation. Placental transfer occurs less readily with drugs possessing a high degree of dissociation or low lipid solubility. The view that the placenta is a barrier to drugs is not correct. The fetus is, to at least some extent, exposed to essentially all drugs taken by the mother (Figure 1–6).

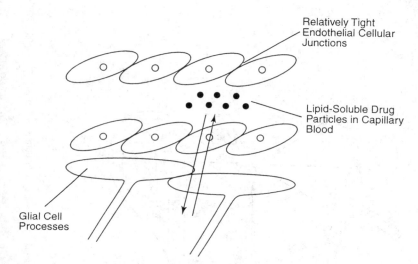

Figure 1–5 Blood-brain barrier. (After Morgan JP. Alcohol and drug abuse, curriculum guide for pharmacology faculty. Rockville, MD: U.S. Department of Health and Human Services, 1985:3.)

DRUG ELIMINATION

Renal Excretion

Drugs are filtered, secreted, and reabsorbed by the kidneys (Figure 1–7).

Filtration: All drugs not bound to plasma proteins are filtered.

Secretion: Some acidic and basic drugs are secreted. This is an active process with transport maxima. Drugs that are secreted usually have short half-lives.

Reabsorption: Drug reabsorption from the renal tubules depends on the percentage of the drug in the nonionized form. Nonionized drug molecules are usually reabsorbed into the systemic circulation. Ionized molecules are not reabsorbed.

Metabolism

Kidneys cannot eliminate lipophilic drug molecules. Lipophilic drugs must first be transformed into ionized, or water-soluble, molecules before the kidney can excrete them. This process is referred to as drug metabolism. Although drug metabolism can occur in most tissues, the liver is the major organ involved in this process. Drug metabolism should not be equated with

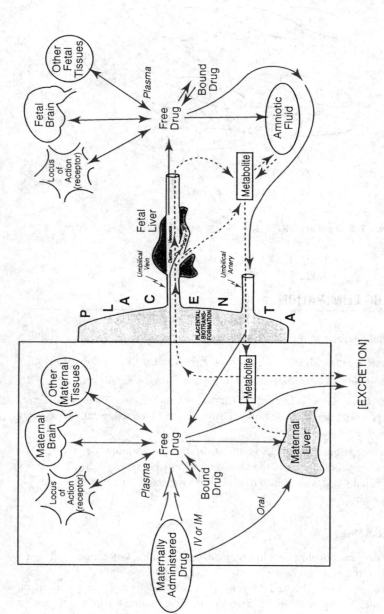

Figure 1–6 Drug distribution in a model of the maternal-placental-fetal unit. (After Mirkin BL. Drug distribution in pregnancy. In: Boreus L, ed. Fetal pharmacology. New York: Raven Press, 1972:22.)

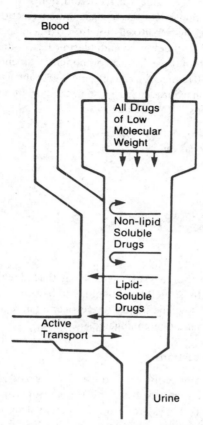

Figure 1–7 Diagrammatic representation of the excretion of drugs by the kidney. (After Brodie BB. Distribution and fate of drugs: therapeutic implications. In: Binns TB, ed. Absorption and distribution of drugs. Edinburgh: E and S Livingston, 1964:201.)

drug inactivation. Although most molecules are inactivated by metabolism, some are activated, and others undergo no change in activity.

Drug metabolism frequently occurs in two separate stages or phases.

Drug $\xrightarrow{\text{Phase I}}$ Introduction of a polar group $\xrightarrow{\text{Phase II}}$ Conjugation of the polar group

Phase I Metabolic Reactions

Phase I involves putting a "handle" (eg, hydroxyl, amine, or carboxyl group) on the drug molecule. If the parent drug already possesses one of these reactive groups, it can be directly conjugated.

Phase I reactions involve oxidation, reduction, or hydrolysis of the drug molecules, with oxidation being the most common reaction. Oxidation reactions are catalyzed by the **mixed-function oxidase enzyme system**, which is mainly found on the smooth endoplasmic reticulum of cells. This enzyme system consists of three distinct components: cytochrome c reductase (cytochrome P-450 reductase), cytochrome P-450, and a phospholipid.

The mixed-function oxidase enzyme system can catalyze a variety of different types of reactions. These include

- Aromatic ring hydroxylation
- Side-chain hydroxylation
- *N*-dealkylation
- *O*-dealkylation
- *S*-dealkylation
- Sulfoxidation
- Desulfuration
- Deamination
- Dehalogenation

If the primary metabolite is sufficiently polar, the kidney can excrete it. If this metabolite is still sufficiently lipophilic to be reabsorbed following glomerular filtration, it will be subject to the second phase of drug metabolism, in which the "handle" is conjugated.

Phase II Metabolic Reactions

Phase II consists of conjugating either the drug or its oxidized metabolite. Conjugation usually involves attaching the conjugating chemical to hydroxyl, amine, or carboxyl group on the parent drug or its primary metabolite formed during phase I. Common conjugating chemicals include

- glucuronic acid (glucuronide conjugates),
- sulfuric acid (sulfate conjugates), and
- glycine (glycine conjugates).

Conjugated metabolites are usually eliminated rapidly by the kidneys.

Figures 1–8 and 1–9 depict the two phases of drug metabolism.

FREQUENTLY USED PHARMACOKINETIC EXPRESSIONS

Bioavailability

Bioavailability refers to the amount of administered drug that reaches the systemic circulation. Two factors can reduce bioavailability: poor absorption and extensive rapid metabolism as the drug passes through the liver or intestine before it reaches the systemic circulation (first-pass metabolism).

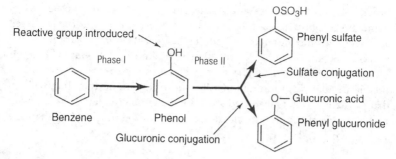

Figure 1–8 Two phases of drug metabolism. (After Gram TE. Metabolism of drugs. In: Craig CR, Stitzel RE, eds. Modern pharmacology. Boston: Little, Brown, 1994:37.)

SUMMARY OF DRUG METABOLISM AND ELIMINATION

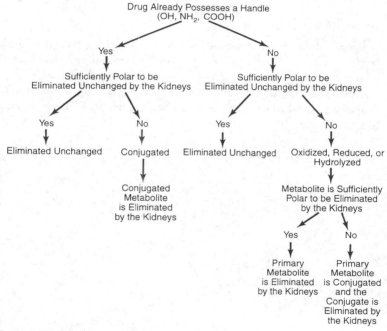

Figure 1–9 Summary of drug metabolism and elimination.

Clearance

Clearance refers to the plasma volume cleared of drug over a given period of time by the kidney (renal clearance), by liver metabolism (hepatic clearance), in the bile (biliary clearance), or by all organs and processes combined (total body clearance). A drug that is rapidly removed by an organ will have a high clearance value. For example, the renal clearance of penicillin G approximates total renal blood flow because the drug is filtered and secreted and not reabsorbed. Therefore, its renal clearance value exceeds 600 mL/minute. A drug that is filtered by the kidney, but not secreted or reabsorbed, will have a renal clearance value that approximates the glomerular filtration rate of 120 mL/minute. If, on the other hand, a drug is extensively reabsorbed into the systemic circulation as it passes down the renal tubules, its clearance value will be much lower than the glomerular filtration rate.

Half-Life

Half-life ($t_{1/2}$) is the time it takes for the plasma concentration, or the amount of drug in the body, to be reduced by 50%. Half-life is expressed in minutes or hours.

Steady State

Drugs are often administered on a regular basis for long periods of time. During the first few doses of a drug its concentration in the body usually increases. Eventually, however, the level of the drug in the body stops increasing and reaches a steady concentration. At this point, the amount of drug being absorbed equals the amount being eliminated. This is referred to as steady state.

Pharmacodynamics: How Drugs Work

DRUG EFFECTS MEDIATED THROUGH DRUG RECEPTORS

Importance to Drug Therapy

Most drugs act in the body by either stimulating or blocking drug receptors. The combination of the drug with the receptor results in a molecular change in the receptor that triggers a chain of events leading to a response within the cell.

Description of a Drug Receptor

A receptor is any cellular macromolecule to which a drug binds to initiate its effects. Although the exact nature of each receptor is not known, it is recognized that each type of receptor shows amazing specificity for the drug or drugs with which it binds.

Agonists

Agonists are chemicals, such as drugs, that interact with a receptor and initiate a cellular reaction. They possess affinity for a receptor, and once attached to the receptor demonstrate intrinsic activity. A cholinergic drug, for example, stimulates muscarinic receptors (see Chapter 4) because it has both **affinity** for these receptors and **intrinsic activity.**

Antagonists

Antagonists have affinity for a receptor, but lack intrinsic activity; therefore, they do not stimulate the receptor. During the time the antagonist occupies the receptor, the drug will block any other chemical from binding to and stimulating the receptor. An anticholinergic, for example, prevents acetylcholine from stimulating muscarinic receptors (see Chapter 4).

Specificity of Drug Receptors

The affinity of a drug for its receptor depends on its chemical structure. Changing the structure of a drug, even slightly, can increase or decrease its affinity for a receptor and significantly modify its pharmacologic effect. For example, epinephrine (see Chapter 5) has affinity for beta$_2$ receptors and causes dilation of bronchioles. The structure of norepinephrine differs from epinephrine only in that the methyl group on epinephrine is replaced by hydrogen on norepinephrine. As a result of this change, norepinephrine has no affinity for beta$_2$ receptors and will not dilate bronchioles.

Effect of Agonists and Antagonists on Drug Receptor Density

Chronic drug therapy can affect receptor density. Long-term treatment with an agonist reduces the number of drug receptors. This is called **down-regulation, tissue tolerance,** or **desensitization**. When this occurs, the effects of the drug diminish. An example of this type of drug-receptor interaction is seen when asthmatic patients receive constant therapy with a beta$_2$ agonist (see Chapter 5) to dilate their bronchioles. As therapy continues, the effect of the drug decreases because of a reduced density of beta$_2$ receptors.

Chronic therapy with an antagonist increases the density of drug receptors (**up-regulation**). For example, long-term treatment with a beta blocker (see Chapter 6) causes an up-regulation of beta receptors. If the beta blocker is suddenly stopped, patients can experience cardiac dysrhythmias through increased sympathetic stimulation of these receptors due to their greater abundance.

DOSE-RESPONSE RELATIONSHIPS

Potency and Intrinsic Activity Of Agonists

The magnitude of a drug response is believed to be a function of the concentration of the drug-receptor complex. Generally, the higher the concentration of the drug at the receptor site, the greater its effect. This occurs up to the point when all receptors have been occupied and a maximum response has been elicited. Increasing the dose of drug administered above this level, and its corresponding concentration at the receptor site, will not result in a further increase in effect.

Figure 2–1 illustrates the mean dose-response curves of three hypothetical drugs.

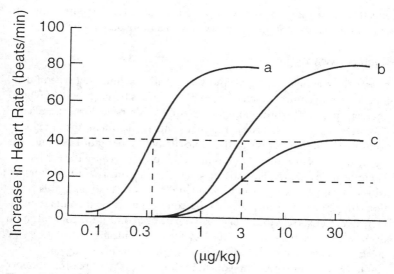

Figure 2–1 Idealized dose-response curves of three agonists (*a,b,c*) that increase heart rate, but differ in potency, maximum effect, or both. Dashed lines indicate 50% of maximum response (horizontal) and individual ED_{50} values (vertical). (After Fleming WW. Mechanisms of drug action. In: Craig CR, Stitzel RE, eds. Modern pharmacology. Boston: Little, Brown, 1994:15.)

Drugs *a* and *b* produce the same maximum effect or response, which is an increase in heart rate of 80 beats per minute. However, the fact that the dose-response curve for drug *a* lies to the left of the curve for drug *b* indicates that drug *a* is more **potent**. The ratio of the potencies for drugs *a* and *b* can be calculated on the basis of their respective ED_{50} values. ED_{50}, is the dose that produces 50% of the maximum response. In the example depicted in Figure 2–1, the difference in potency between *a* and *b* is quantified by the following ratio:

$$ED_{50}b/ED_{50}a.$$

Thus, drug *a* is 10 times more potent than drug *b* (3/0.3).

Drug *c* has a maximum effect that is lower than that of either drug *a* or drug *b*. Drug *c* is said to have a lower **intrinsic activity** than the other two drugs. Drugs *a* and *b* are full agonists with an intrinsic activity of 1; drug *c* is called a **partial agonist** and has an intrinsic activity of 0.5 because its maximum effect is half the maximum effect of *a* or *b*. The potency of drug *c*, however, is the same as that of drug *b*, because both drugs have the same ED_{50} (3 µg/kg).

Therapeutically, it is important not to equate greater potency of a drug with therapeutic superiority as long as it produces the same maximum effect, because one can simply increase the dose of a less potent drug to obtain the identical response observed with a more potent one.

Competitive Antagonism

Competitive antagonism is the most frequently encountered type of drug antagonism in clinical practice. Examples of drugs that exhibit this type of antagonism include antihistamines, H_2-antagonists, beta blockers, and anticholinergics. For these drugs, and many others like them, the antagonist competes with the agonist for the same site on the receptor but unlike the agonist, it does not induce a response on binding because the antagonist has little or no **efficacy**. For most competitive antagonists, the bond formed with the receptor is loose, and the antagonism is **reversible**. In this situation, the antagonism increases as the concentration of the antagonist is increased. Conversely, the antagonism can be overcome if the concentration of the agonist is increased. Figure 2–2 depicts the idealized dose-response curves of an agonist in the absence and presence of increasing doses of an equilibrium-competitive antagonist. In this figure, the increasing presence of the antagonist has shifted the dose-response curves of the agonist to the right. Any level of response is still possible, but greater amounts of the agonist are required to achieve it.

It must be pointed out, however, that the continual shift of the curve to the right, with no change in maximum response as the dose of the antagonist is increased, assumes that very large amounts of the agonist can be delivered to the receptor site. This is usually impossible if the agonist is a

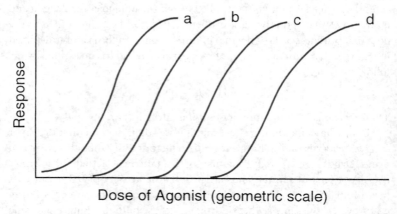

Figure 2–2 Idealized dose-response curves of an agonist in the absence (a) and the presence (b, c, d) of increasing doses of an equilibrium-competitive antagonist. (After Fleming WW. Mechanisms of drug action. In: Craig CR, Stitzel RE, eds. Modern pharmacology. Boston: Little, Brown, 1994:17.)

naturally occurring chemical, such as acetylcholine, epinephrine, or histamine because in this situation, the supply of the agonist is limited. As a result, increasing the concentration of the antagonist at the receptor site will ultimately block the effects of the endogenous agonist.

DRUG EFFECTS NOT MEDIATED THROUGH RECEPTORS

Not all drugs depend on receptors to produce their effects. Antacids, for example, simply depend on neutralizing gastric acid. Cathartics, which work by either irritating the bowel or by drawing water from the blood into the feces by osmosis, also act independent of receptors. It will become apparent throughout the remainder of this book which drug effects depend on drug-receptor interactions and which do not.

Introduction to Autonomic Pharmacology

FUNCTIONS OF THE AUTONOMIC NERVOUS SYSTEM

The autonomic nervous system (Figure 3–1) is composed of the sympathetic and parasympathetic divisions. It functions to innervate

1. smooth muscle,
2. cardiac muscle, and
3. exocrine glands.

It also regulates

1. heart rate,
2. blood pressure,
3. sweat, salivary, and gastric secretions,
4. pupil diameter and eye accommodation,
5. gastrointestinal motility, and
6. diameter of the bronchioles.

DIVISIONS OF THE AUTONOMIC NERVOUS SYSTEM

Common Characteristics of Sympathetic and Parasympathetic Divisions

Each parasympathetic and sympathetic nerve

- originates in the central nervous system (CNS),
- has its activity controlled and integrated by the brain, and
- contains a preganglionic neuron, whose cell of origin lies within the CNS, and a postganglionic neuron, whose cell of origin lies within a

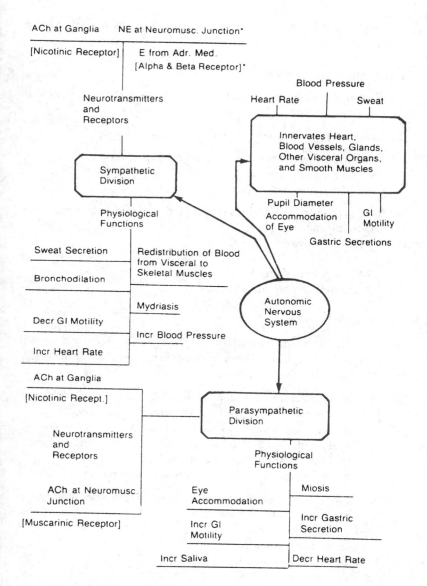

* A few sympathetic nerves, notably those innervating sweat glands, release ACh. In this case the receptors stimulated are muscarinic.

Figure 3–1 Overview of the functions of the sympathetic and parasympathetic divisions of the autonomic nervous system. (Drawing by Ted Johnson.)
ACh = acetylcholine; Decr = decrease; E = epinephrine; GI = gastrointestinal; Incr = increase; NE = norepinephrine.

ganglion outside the CNS. The pre- and postganglionic neurons synapse at a ganglion.

Parasympathetic Division

1. Most preganglionic fibers originate in the midbrain or medulla oblongata of the brain.

2. Ganglia are found close to, or within, innervated organs.

3. A few preganglionic nerves leave the CNS in the sacral portion of the spinal cord. These fibers also synapse with postganglionic nerves close to, or within, the innervated organs.

4. The parasympathetic nervous system carries on many of the mundane day-to-day functions:
   (a) Flow of saliva
   (b) Peristalsis
   (c) Constriction of pupils
   (d) Accommodation for near vision

Sympathetic Division

1. Sympathetic preganglionic fibers begin in the intermediolateral columns of the spinal cord and extend from the first thoracic to the second or third lumbar segments.

2. Once outside the spinal cord, preganglionic fibers synapse with postganglionic nerves at ganglia located in three areas of the body:
   (a) Paravertebral ganglia, which lie on each side of the vertebral column
   (b) Prevertebral ganglia (ie, celiac, superior mesenteric, inferior mesenteric, and aorticorenal ganglia) in the abdominal cavity
   (c) Terminal ganglia near the urinary bladder and rectum

3. Stimulation of the sympathetic nervous system prepares the body to meet stress in the following ways:
   (a) Increasing heart rate
   (b) Elevating cardiac output
   (c) Stimulating intermediary metabolism
   (d) Dilating bronchioles
   (e) Redistributing blood from the GI tract to the skeletal muscles

NEUROTRANSMITTERS

Chemical Transmission of Impulses

Ganglia

Acetylcholine is the neurotransmitter at all autonomic ganglia. Released by preganglionic nerve endings, acetylcholine stimulates **nicotinic receptors** on the postganglionic neurons (Figure 3–2).

Parasympathetic Nerve Endings

Acetylcholine is also the neurotransmitter at all parasympathetic nerve endings. Following its release, acetylcholine stimulates **muscarinic receptors** on the innervated tissue.

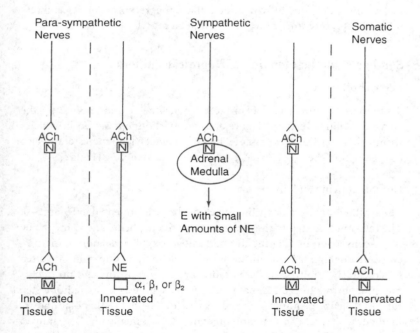

Figure 3–2 Chemical transmission of nerve impulses. ACH = Acetylcholine; NE = norepinephrine; E = Epinephrine; N = nicotinic receptors; M = Muscarinic receptors; α_1 = alpha$_1$ receptors; ß = beta$_1$ or beta$_2$ receptors. (After Johnson GE, Osis M, Hannah KJ. Pharmacology and the nursing practice. 4th ed. Toronto: WB Saunders, 1998:258–260.)

Sympathetic Nerve Endings

Norepinephrine (noradrenaline) is the neurotransmitter released from most sympathetic postganglionic neurons. Once released, it stimulates **alpha₁ receptors** on blood vessels to cause vasoconstriction, or **beta₁ receptors** in the heart to increase both heart rate and force of contraction. **Acetylcholine** is the neurotransmitter released by a few sympathetic postganglionic nerves (eg, sympathetic innervation of the sweat glands), where it stimulates **muscarinic receptors**.

Adrenal Medulla

Epinephrine (adrenaline) is an emergency hormone released by the adrenal medullae. It increases heart rate by stimulating cardiac **beta₁ receptors** and dilates the bronchioles by stimulating **beta₂ receptors**. Adrenaline redistributes blood in the body, shunting it from the peritoneal area to the skeletal muscles. It does this by stimulating **alpha₁ receptors** on visceral vessels and **beta₂ receptors** on vessels in skeletal muscle.

Synthesis and Inactivation of Neurotransmitters

Acetylcholine

Synthesized within nerves from acetylcoenzyme A and choline by the enzyme choline acetylase (Figure 3–3), acetylcholine is stored in vesicles within the nerve until released. The enzyme acetylcholine esterase, also formed within the nerve, rapidly inactivates acetylcholine (Figure 3–4).

Norepinephrine and Epinephrine

The synthesis of norepinephrine and epinephrine is presented in Figure 3–5. The rate-limiting step in the synthesis of norepinephrine and epinephrine is the conversion of tyrosine to dopa (dihydroxyphenylalanine), the precursor of dopamine. Epinephrine, norepinephrine, and dopamine are often called **catecholamines**. In the noradrenergic neurons, the end product is norepinephrine. In the adrenal medulla, the synthesis is carried one step further. An enzyme found in the adrenal medulla, phenylethanolamine-*N*-methyltransferase, converts norepinephrine to epinephrine. The human adrenal medulla contains approximately four times as much epinephrine as norepinephrine. The absence of phenylethanolamine-*N*-methyltransferase in noradrenergic neurons accounts for the absence of significant amounts of epinephrine in noradrenergic neurons.

The final step in the synthesis of norepinephrine, the conversion of dopamine to norepinephrine, takes place within intraneuronal storage vesicles. Norepinephrine is released from noradrenergic nerve endings by

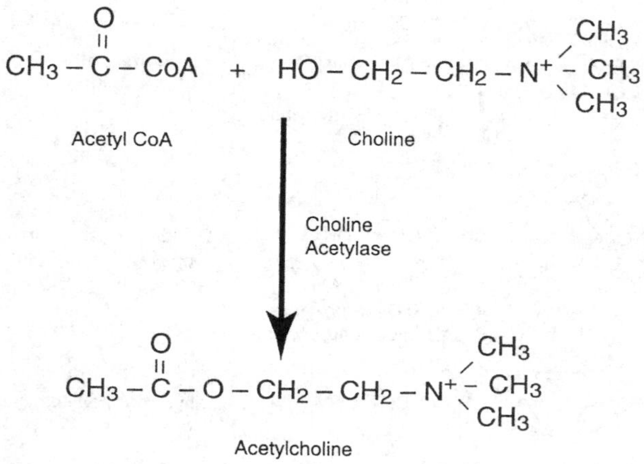

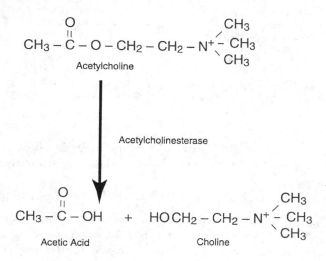

Figure 3–3 Synthesis of acetylcholine. After Johnson GE, Osis M, Hannah KJ. Pharmacology and the nursing practice. 4th ed. Toronto: WB Saunders, 1998:258–260.

Figure 3–4 Inactivation of acetylcholine. After Johnson GE, Osis M, Hannah KJ. Pharmacology and the nursing practice. 4th ed. Toronto: WB Saunders, 1998:258–260.

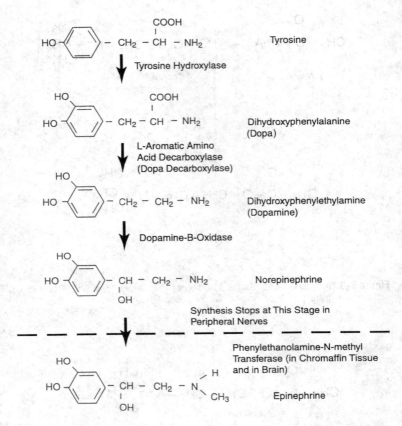

Figure 3-5 Synthesis of norepinephrine and epinephrine. After Johnson GE, Osis M, Hannah KJ. Pharmacology and the nursing practice. 4th ed. Toronto: WB Saunders, 1998:258–260.

action potentials through exocytosis. The norepinephrine contents of entire vesicles are emptied into the synaptic region, where they may interact with adrenergic receptors.

Norepinephrine is removed from the area of the synapse and receptors by

- reuptake into the secreting neuron. Neuronal reuptake is the most important mechanism for terminating the action of released norepinephrine. Following neuronal reuptake, norepinephrine is either stored in vesicles or inactivated by mitochondrial monoamine oxidase (MAO);
- diffusion from the synapse into the circulation and ultimate enzymatic destruction in the liver by MAO or catechol-O-methyltransferase (COMT); and

- active transport of the catecholamine into effector cells (extraneuronal uptake), followed by enzymatic inactivation by COMT.

Figure 3–6 summarizes these processes.

AUTONOMIC RECEPTORS

Cholinergic Receptors

Nicotinic Receptors (so-called because the effects of nicotine in ganglia and on skeletal muscle mimic the actions of acetylcholine)

Found in all autonomic ganglia. Nicotinic receptors are also found on skeletal muscle. However, nicotinic receptors in ganglia are not identical to those on skeletal muscle. Nicotinic receptors in ganglia can be blocked competitively by ganglionic blockers. Ganglionic blockers do not block nicotinic receptors on skeletal muscle; rather, these receptors are blocked by neuromuscular blockers (eg, tubocurarine).

Muscarinic Receptors (so-called because the effects of muscarine on receptors innervated by parasympathetic postganglionic nerves and sympathetic cholinergic nerves mimic the actions of acetylcholine on these receptors)

Found in smooth muscle, cardiac muscle, and exocrine glands innervated by parasympathetic nerves. They are involved in the constriction of bronchioles, slowing of heart rate, increase in GI motility, and secretion of salivary, gastric, and bronchiolar glands. They are also found in sweat glands innervated by the sympathetic nervous system. Muscarinic receptors are also located in the brain. Several subtypes of muscarinic receptors have been detected:

- M_1 receptors are found in various secretory glands.
- M_2 receptors predominate in the myocardium and also appear to be found in smooth muscle.
- M_3 and M_4 receptors are located in smooth muscle and secretory glands.

All subtypes are found in the CNS.

Adrenergic Receptors

Alpha$_1$ Postsynaptic

Found on smooth muscle innervated by sympathetic nerves. Important functions include vasoconstriction of precapillary resistance vessels (arterioles) and capacitance vessels (veins).

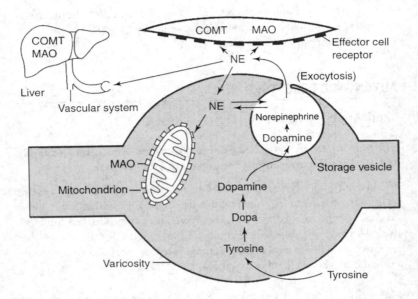

Figure 3–6 Synthesis, storage, release and inactivation of norepinephrine. MAO = monoamine oxidase; COMT = catechol-*O*-methyltransferase; NE = norepinephrine. (After Fleming WW. Introduction to the autonomic nervous system. In: Craig CR, Stitzel RE, eds. Modern Pharmacology. Boston: Little, Brown, 1994;108.)

Alpha$_2$ Presynaptic

Found on adrenergic nerve terminals. They are responsible for reducing the release of norepinephrine from sympathetic nerves.

Beta$_1$ Postsynaptic

Found on postsynaptic effector cells, especially in the heart. They are responsible for the sympathetically mediated increase in heart rate and force of contraction. They are also found on fat cells where they are responsible for the sympathetically mediated increase in lipolysis. Beta$_1$ receptors also mediate the release of renin.

Beta$_2$ Postsynaptic

Found on bronchioles, where they mediate sympathetic bronchodilation. They are located on precapillary resistance vessels (arterioles) in skeletal muscle where they mediate vasodilation. Beta$_2$ receptors relax the bladder and decrease intestinal motility.

4

Cholinergic and Anticholinergic Drugs

CHOLINERGIC DRUGS (Figure 4–1)

Drugs Directly Stimulating Cholinergic Receptors

Rationale for Directly Acting Cholinergics

Acetylcholine has little value as a drug because

- it is rapidly metabolized by acetylcholinesterase and serum cholinesterase, and
- it stimulates both muscarinic and nicotinic receptors.

Directly acting cholinergics have partially overcome these limitations. These drugs

- are resistant to cholinesterase hydrolysis and have a longer duration of action than acetylcholine, and
- show some selectivity for muscarinic receptors. However, only bethanechol appears to completely lack nicotinic agonist effects (Table 4–1).

General Uses for Directly Acting Cholinergics

In the Eye

Carbachol and pilocarpine are instilled in the eye to stimulate circular muscles in the iris to produce miosis. This action increases the drainage of the aqueous humor through the canals of Schlemm and lowers intraocular pressure in glaucoma. Carbachol and pilocarpine can also produce hyperemia and aching eyes and head. Refer to Figure 4–2 and Table 4–2 for a review of the autonomic pharmacology of the eye.

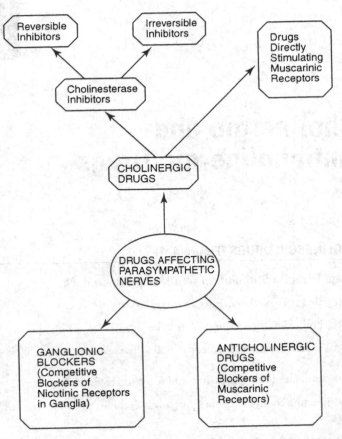

Figure 4–1 Diagrammatic representation of the types of drugs affecting the parasympathetic nervous system. (Drawing by Ted Johnson.)

Systemically

Carbachol and bethanechol stimulate muscarinic receptors in the bladder and intestinal tract. They are used to treat postoperative intestinal atony, postoperative urinary retention, and neurogenic atony of the bladder. Stimulation of muscarinic receptors in the heart can be used to treat paroxysmal tachycardia. The systemic administration of these drugs also increases gastric acid secretion, constricts bronchioles, increases salivary and sweat secretion, and dilates blood vessels. Adverse effects include sweating, salivation, flushing, decreased blood pressure, nausea, abdominal pain, diarrhea, bronchospasm, cardiac arrest, and circulatory collapse.

Table 4–1

Comparative Pharmacologic Properties of Some Directly Acting Cholinergics

Chemical	Suscept-ibility to cholin-esterases	Muscarinic Effects				Nico-tinic Effects
		Cardio-vascular	GI and Bladder	Eye	Sweat	
Acetylcholine	+++	++	++	+	+	++
Carbachol	-	+++	++	+	+	+++
Bethanechol	-	±	+++	++	+	-
Pilocarpine	-	±	++	+++	++	+

Cholinesterase Inhibitors (Anticholinesterases)

Cholinesterase inhibitors potentiate and prolong the effects of acetylcholine released by neurons at

- neuromuscular junctions,
- adrenal medullae,
- autonomic ganglia,
- cholinergic synapses of the autonomic nervous system (ie, postganglionic parasympathetic nerves and a few postganglionic sympathetic nerves), and
- cholinergic synapses in the central nervous system.

Table 4–3 summarizes the effects of cholinesterase inhibitors.

Table 4–2

Summary of Autonomic Innervation of the Eye

Part of the Eye	Innervation	Receptors	Effects
Iris	Parasympathetic to circular muscle	Muscarinic	Constriction of pupil (miosis)
	Sympathetic to longitudinal muscle	Alpha$_1$	Dilation of pupil (mydriasis)
Ciliary Body	Parasympathetic to circular muscle	Muscarinic	Constriction of sphincter permitting accommodation

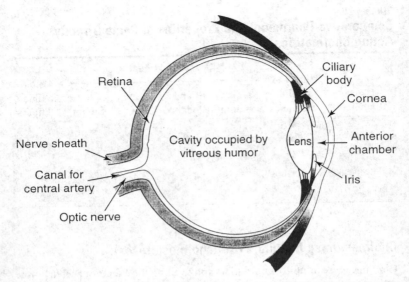

Figure 4–2 Autonomic innervation of the eye. (After Johnson GE, Osis M, Hannah KJ. Pharmacology and the nursing practice. 4th ed. Toronto: WB Saunders, 1998:265.)

Anticholinesterase drugs can be divided into:

- Reversible cholinesterase inhibitors:
  - ◆ Carbamates (neostigmine, pyridostigmine, physostigmine, ambenonium, and demecarium), and
  - ◆ Quaternary nitrogen compounds (edrophonium) and
- Irreversible cholinesterase inhibitors:
  - ◆ Phosphates (echothiophate), and
  - ◆ Fluorophosphates (isoflurophate)

Figures 4–3 and 4–4 provide the structures of reversible and irreversible cholinesterase inhibitors.

Mechanism of Action of Reversible Cholinesterase Inhibitors (Figure 4–5)

Carbamates

$$R_2\text{-N-C-O-R}$$

Bind to the esteratic site on the cholinesterase molecule preventing acetylcholine from attaching to the enzyme.

Table 4–3
Effects of Cholinesterase Inhibitors

Body Organ	Effect of Cholinesterase Inhibitor
Skin	Increased sweat
Eye	Lacrimation, miosis, blurred vision, spasm of accommodation
Digestive tract	Salivation; increased gastric, pancreatic and intestinal secretions; increased gut tone and motility (abdominal cramps, vomiting, diarrhea, and defecation)
Urinary tract	Urinary frequency and incontinence
Respiratory tract	Increased bronchial secretions, bronchoconstriction, weakness or paralysis of respiratory muscles
Skeletal muscle	Fasciculations, weakness, depolarizing block and paralysis
Cardiovascular system	Bradycardia (due to muscarinic effects), decreased cardiac output, hypotension These may be counterbalanced by ganglionic stimulation at the adrenal medullae and the release of increased amounts of adrenaline
Central nervous system	Tremor, anxiety, restlessness, disrupted concentration and memory, confusion, sleep disturbances, desynchronization of electroencephalogram, convulsions, coma, circulatory and respiratory depression

Quaternary Nitrogen Drugs
R-N$^+$-(R)$_3$

Attach to the anionic site on the cholinesterase molecule, preventing acetylcholine from binding to this site.

General Uses for Reversible Cholinesterase Inhibitors

In the Eye

Physostigmine and demecarium are instilled in the eye to produce miosis and increase drainage of the aqueous humor in the treatment of glaucoma.

Systemically

Neostigmine is used to increase muscarinic stimulation in the intestine and bladder in the prophylaxis or treatment of intestinal atony and urinary retention. It is also used to reverse the effects of competitive neuromuscular

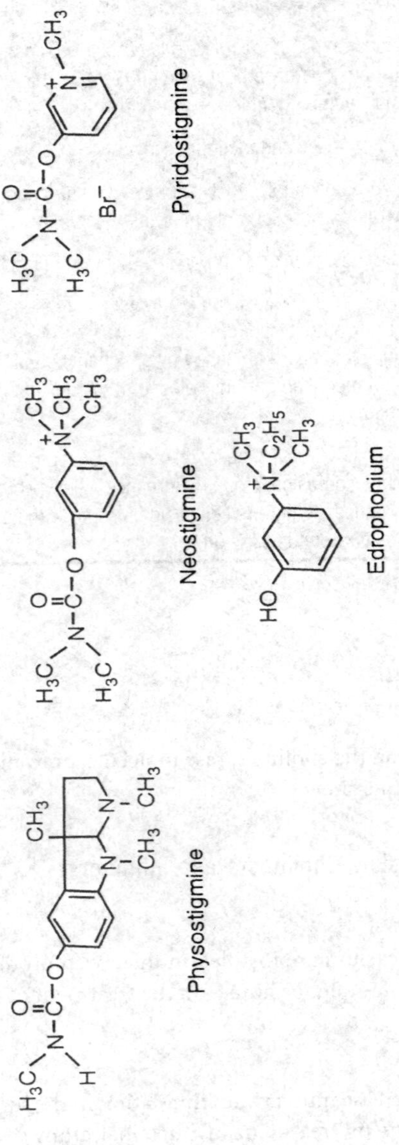

Figure 4–3 Representatives of reversible cholinesterase inhibitors.

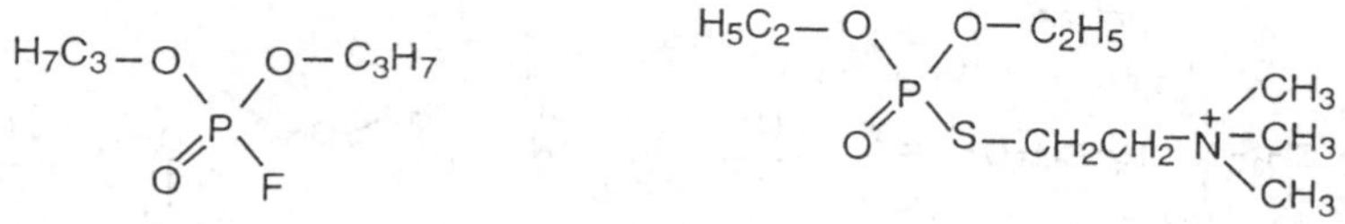

Figure 4–4 Representatives of irreversible cholinesterase inhibitors

blockers (see Chapter 7). Along with pyridostigmine and ambenonium, neostigmine is also used to increase stimulation of nicotinic receptors in the treatment of myasthenia gravis.

Mechanism of Action of Irreversible Cholinesterase Inhibitors

Phosphates or Fluorophosphates

Irreversible inhibitors of cholinesterase phosphorylate the esteratic site on the cholinesterase molecule. The phosphorylated enzyme is a stable complex. Recovery from the effects of an irreversible inhibitor usually depends on the synthesis of new cholinesterase molecules (Figure 4–6).

General Uses for Irreversible Cholinesterase Inhibitors

In the Eye

Instilled in the eye, these drugs produce marked miosis. They are used when other miotics fail to decrease the intraocular pressure in glaucoma. Because they are also absorbed into the systemic circulation, irreversible cholinesterase inhibitors may also produce systemic cholinergic stimulation. Other adverse effects include cataracts, spasm of accommodation, and cysts of the iris.

ANTICHOLINERGIC DRUGS (See Figure 4–1)

Mechanism of Action

Anticholinergic drugs competitively block muscarinic receptors, inhibiting all parasympathetic functions and sympathetic cholinergic activity (eg, sweat).

Figure 4–7 provides the chemical structures of several anticholinergics. These drugs compete with acetylcholine for muscarinic receptors because

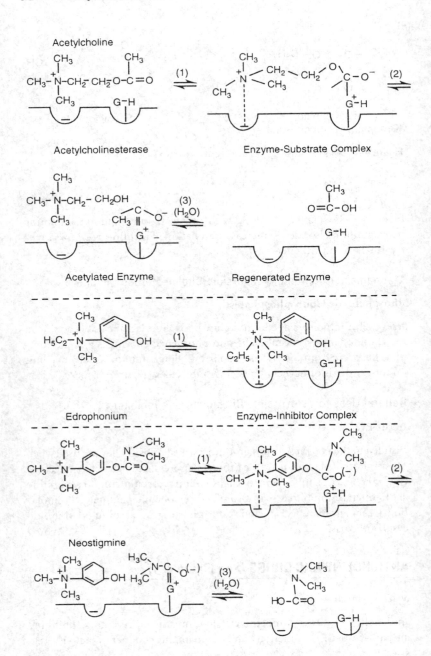

Figure 4–5 Interaction of acetylcholine, edrophonium, and neostigmine with the cholinesterase molecule, demonstrating how the latter two chemicals prevent the attachment of acetylcholine to the enzyme.

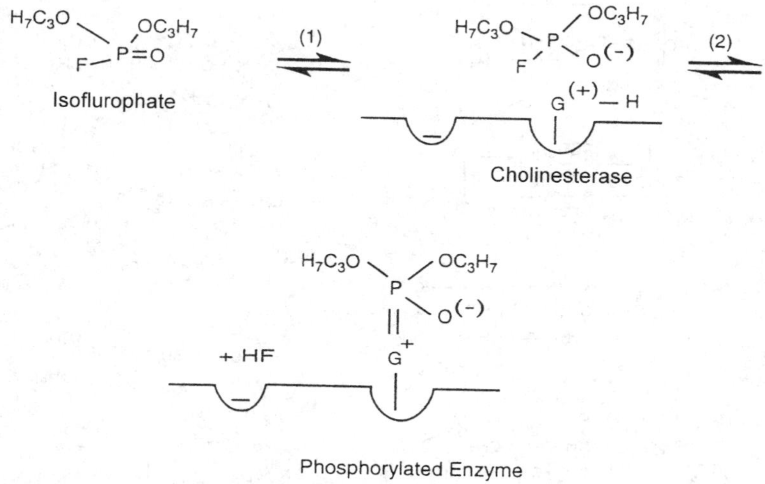

Figure 4–6 Interaction of isoflurophate with a cholinesterase molecule.

the intra-atomic distance between the esteratic group and the nitrogen on each anticholinergic is the same as on acetylcholine.

General Uses for Anticholinergic Drugs

In the Eye

Anticholinergics, such as homatropine, eucatropine, cyclopentolate, and tropicamide, block muscarinic receptors on the circular muscle of the iris. As a result, sympathetic stimulation of the alpha$_1$ receptors on the longitudinal muscles of the iris can act unopposed by cholinergic stimulation and dilate the pupil (mydriasis). Anticholinergics also block muscarinic receptors on the ciliary body and inhibit accommodation for near vision (cycloplegia). Anticholinergics are used for intraocular examination, intraocular surgery, estimation of errors of refraction, and as a provocative test for angle-closure glaucoma.

Systemically

Anticholinergics reduce muscarinic stimulation throughout the body. They are used for blocking bronchiolar secretion, which aids in anesthesia; inhibiting GI secretion and activity, which may facilitate the treatment of peptic ulcers and irritable bowel syndrome; and decreasing vagal tone to the heart, which can be of value in carotid sinus syndrome. The adverse effects of systemically administered anticholinergics include mydriasis, cyclople-

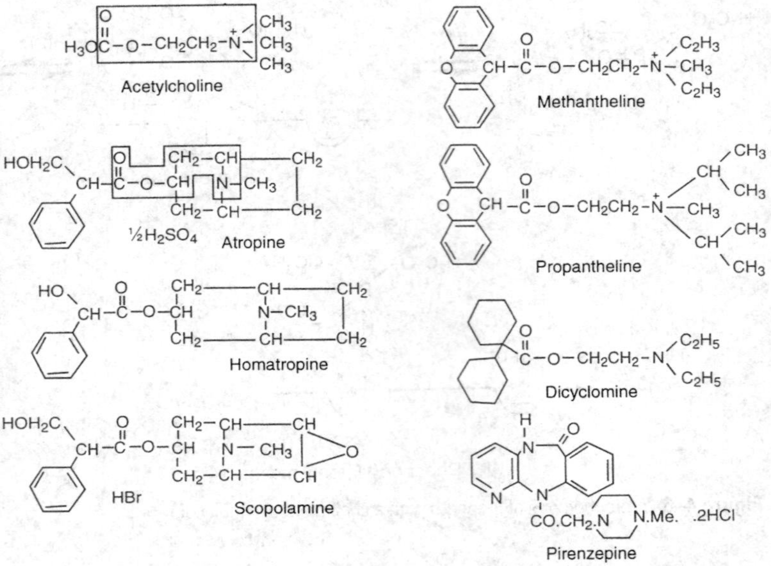

Figure 4–7 Structures of acetylcholine and several anticholinergics, showing structural similarity between acetylcholine and atropine.

gia, dryness of the mouth, flushing, tachycardia, irritability, thirst, fever, ataxia, confusion, somnolence, hallucinations, and delirium.

GANGLIONIC BLOCKERS (See Figure 4–1)

Mechanism of Action

Ganglionic blockers competitively inhibit acetylcholine from stimulating nicotinic receptors in sympathetic and parasympathetic ganglia. Examples of ganglionic blocking drugs include hexamethonium, mecamylamine, chorisondamine, and trimethaphan.

Uses

Ganglionic blockers are rarely used in medicine because they inhibit all autonomic functions. Their effects include hypotension, tachycardia, dryness of the mouth and skin, constipation, and cycloplegia.

5

Adrenergic Drugs (Sympathomimetics)

Prior to beginning this chapter, it would be beneficial to review the synthesis and inactivation of norepinephrine and epinephrine (see Figures 3–5 and 3–6), as well as the functions of alpha and beta receptors (pages 26 and 27 and Figure 5–1).

Adrenergic drugs may act

- directly by stimulating adrenergic receptors, or
- indirectly by releasing norepinephrine from sympathetic neurons (Figure 5–2).

DIRECTLY ACTING ADRENERGICS

May Stimulate

1. Alpha$_1$ (α_1)-adrenergic receptors
2. Beta (β)-adrenergic receptors
3. α_1- and β-adrenergic receptors
4. Dopamine receptors

Figure 5–3 presents the structure of epinephrine, norepinephrine, dopamine, and isoproterenol. The first two demand immediate attention because most adrenergic drugs are designed to mimic the properties of one, or both, of these naturally occurring compounds. Table 5–1 and Figure 5–4 compare the activities of epinephrine and norepinephrine.

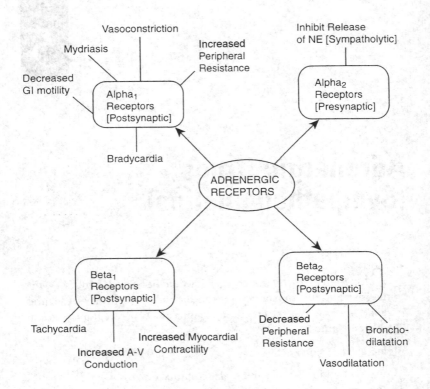

Figure 5–1 Actions mediated by adrenergic receptors. (Drawing by Ted Johnson.) NE = norepinephrine; GI = gastrointestinal.

DIFFERENCES BETWEEN EPINEPHRINE AND NOREPINEPHRINE

Epinephrine: Emergency Hormone Secreted in Stress

1. Increases cardiac output (CO) (β_1)
2. Redistributes blood from viscera to skeletal muscles by constricting precapillary resistance vessels (arterioles) in the abdomen (α_1) and dilating precapillary resistance vessels in skeletal muscles (β_2)
3. Maintains venous return by constricting capacitance vessels (veins) (α_1)
4. Dilates bronchioles (β_2)

Norepinephrine: Sympathetic Neurotransmitter Responsible for Routine Cardiovascular Control

1. Increases heart rate (β_1) when released by cardiac accelerator nerves

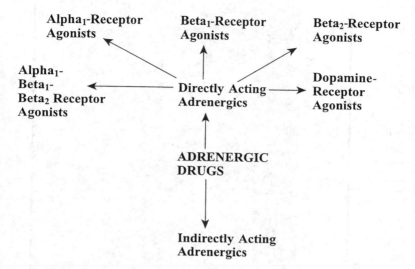

Figure 5–2 Classification of adrenergic drugs.

2. Decreases heart rate when infused because the increase in peripheral resistance reflexly stimulates the vagus, overcoming the direct β_1 stimulation produced by norepinephrine

3. Maintains peripheral resistance by constricting precapillary resistance vessels (α_1)

4. Maintains venous return and prevents orthostatic hypotension by constricting capacitance vessels (α_1)

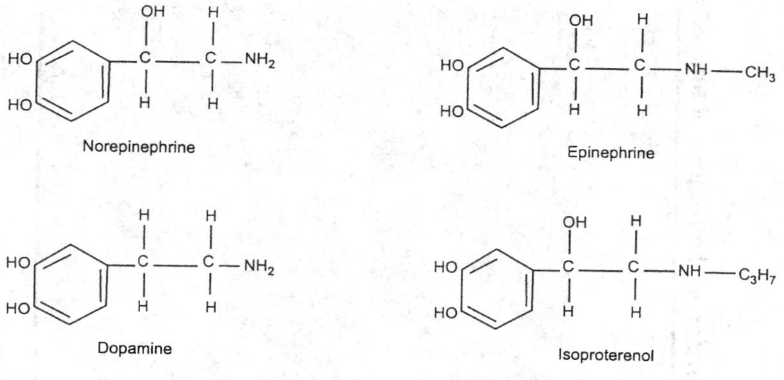

Figure 5–3 Structures of norepinephrine, epinephrine, dopamine, and isoproterenol.

Table 5–1
Comparison of the Actions of Infused Epinephrine and Norepinephrine

	Heart Rate and Force of Contraction	Peripheral Resistance	Venous Return	Bronchioles
Epinephrine	Increases both heart rate and force of contraction; a β_1-mediated effect	Decreases peripheral resistance. Stimulates α_1-receptors on arterioles in the abdomen, and β_2-receptors on arterioles in skeletal muscle, with the latter effect being greater	Increases venous return due to α_1-receptor stimulation of the veins (capacitance vessels)	Dilates bronchioles, due to β_2-receptor stimulation
Norepinephrine	Decreases heart rate. The direct β_1-receptor stimulation on the heart is more than counterbalanced by reflex vagal bradycardia, resulting from an increase in peripheral resistance by α_1-receptor stimulation of the arterioles	Increases peripheral resistance, due to α_1-receptor stimulation of arterioles (precapillary resistance vessels)	Increases venous return due to α_1-stimulation of the veins (capacitance vessels)	No major effect

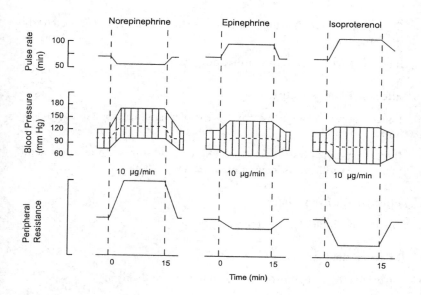

Figure 5–4 Comparison of the effects of infused norepinephrine, epinephrine, and isoproterenol on pulse rate, blood pressure, and peripheral resistance. (After Allwood MJ, Cobbold AE, Ginsburg J. Peripheral vascular effects of noradrenaline, isopropylnoradrenaline and dopamine. Br Med Bull 1963; 19:132.)

1. α_1-, β_1-, and β_2- Receptor Agonists (Epinephrine/Adrenaline)

Effect on Blood Vessels and Vascular Resistance

Constrict arterioles (precapillary resistance vessels) in skin, mucous membranes, kidneys, and splanchnic beds (α_1-receptors).

Dilate arterioles in skeletal muscles (β_2-receptors).

Small doses reduce total peripheral resistance (TPR) because the decrease in PR in skeletal muscles exceeds the increase in PR in cutaneous and mucous membranes, kidneys, and splanchnic area.

Large doses increase TPR due to a generalized α_1 stimulation.

Increase venous return due to α_1 stimulation of veins (capacitance vessels).

Effect on the Heart

Increase cardiac contractility (β_1-receptors).

Increase heart rate (β_1), unless an increase in TPR from high doses reflexly slows the heart.

Increase stroke volume and cardiac output.

Effect on Blood Pressure

Ranges from no change to a moderate increase in mean pressure with low doses.

Increase systolic pressure. Decrease diastolic pressure with low doses and increase diastolic pressure with higher doses.

Effect on the Bronchioles

Dilate bronchioles (β_2-receptors).

Effect on the Eye

Mydriasis (α_1-receptors on the radial muscles of the iris).

Epinephrine decreases intraocular pressure in glaucoma by increasing drainage of aqueous humor, possibly due to vasodilation of conjunctival blood vessels.

Additional Effects

Decrease in GI motility and tone (β_2-receptor stimulation).

Relaxation of uterus (β_2-receptor stimulation).

Relaxation of urinary bladder (β_2-receptor stimulation).

Increase in lipolysis (β_1-receptors) and glycogenolysis (β_2-receptor stimulation).

Uses

Epinephrine is used to

- treat bronchospasm,
- treat hypersensitivity reactions,
- prolong action of local anesthetics,
- treat cardiac arrest, and
- treat open-angle glaucoma.

Adverse Effects

Anxiety, fear, tenseness, restlessness, headache, tremor, weakness, dizziness, pallor, respiratory difficulty, palpitations.

2. α₁-Receptor Agonists (Norepinephrine/Noradrenaline/ Levarterenol, Methoxamine, and Phenylephrine)

Effect on Blood Vessels and Vascular Resistance

Constrict arterioles (precapillary resistance vessels) in skin, mucous membranes, skeletal muscles, kidneys, and splanchnic beds.

Increase TPR.

Increase venous tone.

Effect on the Heart

Decrease heart rate as a result of an increase in TPR and reflex vagal stimulation.

Effect on Blood Pressure

Increase in mean, diastolic, and systolic pressures.

No change in pulse pressure.

Additional Effects

Mydriasis, due to stimulation of radial muscles of the iris.

Uses

(a) Systemic (all of the above drugs) — (a) maintenance of blood pressure (BP) in acute hypotensive states, (b) surgical and nonsurgical trauma, (c) central vasomotor depression, and (d) hemorrhage.

Phenylephrine in nose — vasoconstriction and decongestion in the common cold; treatment of vasomotor and allergic rhinitis and sinusitis.

Phenylephrine in eye — relief of conjunctivitis; production of mydriasis during refraction, ophthalmic examination, or diagnostic procedures.

Adverse Effects

Systemic—bradycardia, ventricular extrasystoles and tachycardia (from phenylephrine), headache, local necrosis.

Phenylephrine in nose or eye—burning, stinging, dryness of mucosa, palpitations, tachycardia, arrhythmias, increase in BP, headache, blurred vision, central nervous system (CNS) depression.

3. β-Receptor Agonists

Beta-adrenergic drugs may be divided into the following groups (Figure 5–5):

- β_1-, β_2- Receptor agonists (isoproterenol)
- β_1-Receptor agonists (dobutamine)
- β_2-Receptor agonists used to dilate bronchioles (albuterol/salbutamol, fenoterol, salmeterol, terbutaline)
- β_2-Receptor agonists used to dilate peripheral arterioles (nylidrin)
- β_2-Receptor agonists used to decrease both the frequency and intensity of uterine contractions (ritodrine)

A. β_1-, β_2-Receptor Agonists (Isoproterenol)

Effect on the Heart

Increase heart rate and force of contraction (a β_1-mediated effect).

Effect on the Bronchioles

Dilate bronchioles (a β_2-mediated effect).

Effect on Blood Vessels

Dilate blood vessels (a β_2-mediated effect).

Uses

Isoproterenol is used to

- treat low cardiac output,
- dilate bronchioles, and
- treat asthma.

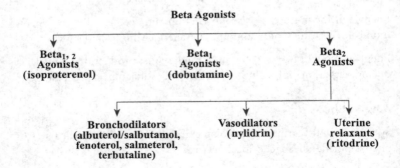

Figure 5–5 Classification of β-agonists.

Adverse Effects

Refractory bronchospasm, palpitations, tachycardia, cardiac arrhythmias, cardiac arrest, hypotension, headache, nausea, tremor, insomnia.

B. β₁-Receptor Agonists (Dobutamine)

Effect on the Heart

Increases both heart rate and force of contraction, with a greater effect on contractile force.

Effect on Renal Vessels

Does not stimulate dopamine receptors on renal vasculature, and, therefore, it does not dilate renal vessels.

Uses

Is used to treat cardiac decompensation due to depressed contractility from organic heart disease or surgical procedures. The major advantage of dobutamine over other sympathomimetics is that it increases cardiac output with a minimal effect on heart rate.

Adverse Effects

Tachycardia, angina, cardiac arrhythmias, headache, hypertension, nausea, vomiting.

C. β₂-Receptor Agonist Bronchodilators (Albuterol/Salbutamol, Fenoterol, Salmeterol, Terbutaline)

Actions

Dilate bronchioles.

Increase forced expiratory volume in one second (FEV_1).

Increase forced expiratory flow (FEF).

Produce tachycardia in higher doses.

Uses

Relief of bronchospasm.

Treatment of chronic bronchitis.

Treatment of bronchopulmonary disorders in which bronchospasm is a complicating factor.

Adverse Effects

Headache, dizziness, nausea, tremor, palpitations.

Advantages over Nonselective β-Receptor Agonists, such as Isoproterenol

Greater Selectivity For Beta₂ Receptors

These drugs are more selective in their ability to preferentially stimulate β_2-receptors. Nonselective β-agonists, such as isoproterenol, stimulate both β_1- and β_2-receptors. As a result, nonselective beta agonists increase heart rate, while they dilate bronchioles. In normal therapeutic doses, selective β_2-agonists dilate bronchioles, while producing little tachycardia (Figure 5–6).

Oral Effectiveness

Isoproterenol is not effective orally. Most β_2-agonists can be given orally or by inhalation.

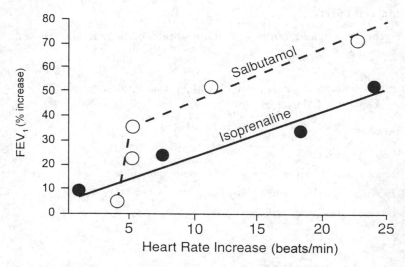

Figure 5–6 Comparison of isoproterenol (isoprenaline) and salbutamol/albuterol demonstrating the significant increase in FEV₁ with minimal effects on heart rate with the latter compound when lower doses are used. (After Paterson JW. Human pharmacology: comparison of intravenous isoprenaline and salbutamol in salbutamol in asthmatic patients. Postgrad Med J 1971; 47(March Suppl.):39.)

Longer Duration of Action

Isoproterenol has a short duration of action (approximately 2 to 3 hours). The β_2-agonists have longer durations of action and are more convenient for the patient.

D. β_2-Vasodilators (Nylidrin)

Actions

Nylidrin stimulates β_2-receptors and produces peripheral vasodilatation of arteries and arterioles in skeletal muscle. It also has positive inotropic effects, reflecting some β_1-stimulation.

Uses

Possible benefit in the treatment of peripheral vascular disease.

Adverse Effects

Trembling, nervousness, weakness, nausea, vomiting, dizziness, palpitations, postural hypotension.

E. β_2-Uterine Relaxants (Ritodrine)

Actions

Ritodrine stimulates β_2-receptors to decrease both the frequency and intensity of uterine contractions. To a lesser degree, ritodrine stimulates β_1-receptors, resulting in a dose-related tachycardia.

Uses

Management of preterm labor (ie, > 20 and < 37 weeks gestation) in suitable patients who have intact amniotic membranes, cervical dilatation up to 4 cm, and less than 80% cervical effacement.

Adverse Effects

Result mainly from β-receptor adrenergic stimulation. These include: tachycardia; increase in systolic and decrease in diastolic pressure; rise in blood glucose, insulin, and free fatty acids; and a decrease in serum potassium. Ritodrine can also cause palpitations, tremor, nausea, vomiting, hyperglycemia, headaches, nervousness, anxiety, malaise, chest pains and tightness, and erythema. Fetal tachycardia, neonatal hypoglycemia, and hypocalcemia have been reported. Fetus can also be affected by maternal ketoacidosis.

4. Dopamine Agonists (Dopamine)

Actions

Stimulates specific dopamine receptors.

Stimulates α_1- and β_1-receptors.

Releases norepinephrine from adrenergic nerves endings.

Produces a dose-dependent cardiovascular response:

- Low doses of dopamine dilate the renal, mesenteric, coronary, and intracerebral vascular beds, with little effect on the heart. The vasodilatation is mediated by specific dopamine receptors.
  - Stimulation of D_1-receptors on blood vessels, and certain other peripheral sites, results in vasodilation, natriuresis, and diuresis.
  - Stimulation of D_2-receptors on ganglia, the adrenal cortex, and within the cardiovascular centers of the CNS produces hypotension, bradycardia, and renal vasodilatation.

- Moderately higher doses of dopamine increase the rate and contractile force of the heart and increase cardiac output. This action is mediated by stimulation of β_1-receptors and the release of norepinephrine. Dopamine increases the force of contraction more than heart rate. As a result, it produces a smaller increase in oxygen demand by the heart than do drugs, such as isoproterenol, that only stimulate β-receptors.

- Higher doses of dopamine stimulate the heart and cause an α_1-receptor-mediated vasoconstriction in most vascular beds.

- Still higher doses of dopamine can constrict the renal and mesenteric beds.

Uses

Treatment of cardiogenic shock, which may be due to myocardial infarction or congestive heart failure.

Treatment of septic shock.

Dopamine has the advantage of increasing cardiac output, while dilating renal blood vessels and improving blood flow to the kidneys.

Adverse Effects

Tachycardia, angina pectoris, cardiac arrhythmias, headache, hypertension, nausea, vomiting, constriction of renal vessels (produced by high doses).

INDIRECTLY ACTING ADRENERGICS (EPHEDRINE)

Actions

Peripheral actions of ephedrine depend primarily on the release of norepinephrine from noradrenergic nerves. Ephedrine increases systolic and diastolic blood pressure, the contractile force of the heart, and cardiac output.

Ephedrine also directly stimulates β_2-adrenergic receptors, accounting for its bronchodilating effects.

Ephedrine crosses the blood-brain barrier and stimulates the CNS.

Uses

Treatment of nasal congestion and bronchial asthma.

Used in the eye as a mydriatic.

Adverse Effects

Similar to epinephrine.

6

Antiadrenergic Drugs (Sympatholytics)

CLASSIFICATION OF ANTIADRENERGIC DRUGS (FIGURE 6–1)

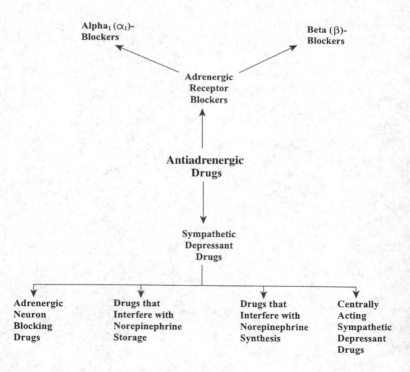

Figure 6–1 Classification of antiadrenergic drugs.

Sympathetic Depressant Drugs (Figure 6–2)

Depress the sympathetic nervous system by either

1. blocking adrenergic neurons (guanethidine),
2. interfering with norepinephrine storage (reserpine),
3. inhibiting the synthesis of norepinephrine (α-methyltyrosine), or
4. preventing norepinephrine release within the CNS (clonidine, α-methyldopa).

Adrenergic Receptor Blockers (Figure 6–3)

Inhibit various aspects of sympathetic function by blocking either

1. α_1-receptors,
2. β-receptors, or
3. α_1- and β-receptors.

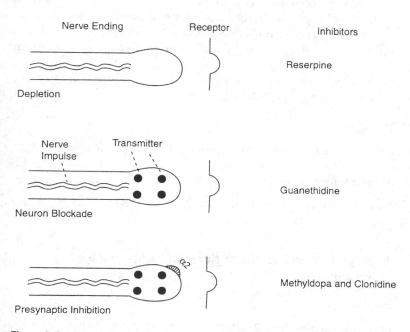

Figure 6–2 Mechanisms of action of sympathetic depressant drugs. (After Spector S, Pradhan SN. Drugs affecting catecholaminergic neurotransmisson. In: Pradhan SN, Maikel RP, Dutta SN, eds. Pharmacology in medicine: principles and practice. Bethesda: SP Press International, 1986:103.)

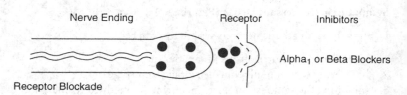

Figure 6–3 Action of alpha₁ and beta blockers. (After Spector S, Pradhan SN. Drugs affecting catecholaminergic neurotransmission. In: Pradhan SN, Maikel RP, Dutta SN, eds. Pharmacology in medicine; principles and practice. Bethesda: SP Press International, 1986:103.)

SYMPATHETIC DEPRESSANT DRUGS

1. Adrenergic Neuron Blocking Drugs (Guanethidine)

Actions

Guanethidine accumulates in adrenergic neurons and disrupts the process by which action potentials trigger the release of stored norepinephrine.

Guanethidine also reduces blood pressure. It dilates arterioles, decreasing peripheral resistance, and it also dilates veins, decreasing venous return and reducing cardiac output.

Renal, splanchnic, and cerebral blood flow all fall in proportion to the reduction in cardiac output.

Uses

Guanethidine is used in the treatment of essential hypertension.

Adverse Effects

Postural hypotension, weakness, fluid retention, heart failure in patients with depressed myocardial function, diarrhea.

2. Drugs That Interfere with Norepinephrine Storage (Reserpine)

Actions

Reserpine reduces the uptake of norepinephrine by intraneuronal vesicles. Much of the norepinephrine released from adrenergic nerves is reabsorbed by the neurons and stored in intraneuronal vesicles. Storage in these vesicles is essential to protect norepinephrine from monoamine oxidase metabolism. Because reserpine inhibits the uptake of norepinephrine by the intraneuronal vesicles, much of the reabsorbed norepinephrine is metabolized within the nerve. As a result, norepinephrine levels within the sympathetic nerves fall and sympathetic transmission is reduced.

Reserpine

- decreases blood pressure,
- slows heart rate,
- reduces cardiac output,
- decreases venous return,
- produces CNS depression,
- increases gastrointestinal tone and motility, and
- increases gastric acid secretion.

Uses

Reserpine is used to treat mild to moderate hypertension.

Adverse Effects

Depression, nightmares, abdominal cramps, diarrhea, flushing, nasal congestion, postural hypotension.

3. Drugs that Interfere with Norepinephrine Synthesis (α-Methyltyrosine/Metyrosine)

Actions

Metyrosine blocks the action of tyrosine hydroxylase and prevents the conversion of tyrosine to dopa, the rate-limiting step in the synthesis of the catecholamines dopamine, norepinephrine, and epinephrine (see Chapter 3).

Uses

Metyrosine is useful for the preoperative treatment of pheochromocytoma and for long-term therapy when surgery is not feasible.

Adverse Effects

Sedation, extrapyramidal effects, diarrhea, nasal congestion, dryness of mouth.

4. Centrally Acting Sympathetic Depressant Drugs (α-Methyldopa, Clonidine)

A. α-Methyldopa

Actions

α-Methyldopa rapidly enters the brain where it accumulates in noradrenergic nerves. Within noradrenergic nerves, α-methyldopa is first converted to α-methyldopamine by dopa decarboxylase and then to α-methylnorepinephrine by dopamine β-oxidase (Figure 6–4). α-Methylnorepinephrine replaces norepinephrine within the central sympathetic neurons and is released in place of norepinephrine by sympathetic stimulation. When α-methylnorepinephrine is released, it stimulates α$_2$-adrenergic receptors in the medulla oblongata to reduce subsequent central sympathetic outflow.

α-Methyldopa also reduces blood pressure. In younger patients with uncomplicated hypertension, it reduces vascular resistance without causing much change in cardiac output. In older patients, α-methyldopa may act primarily by dilating veins, thereby reducing preload and cardiac output.

Uses

α-Methyldopa is used to treat essential hypertension. Because plasma volume increases during prolonged treatment, α-methyldopa is usually combined with a diuretic.

Adverse Effects

Sedation, headache, postural hypotension, bradycardia, edema, drug fever, hepatic dysfunction, hemolytic anemia, impotence, lactation, nausea, vomiting.

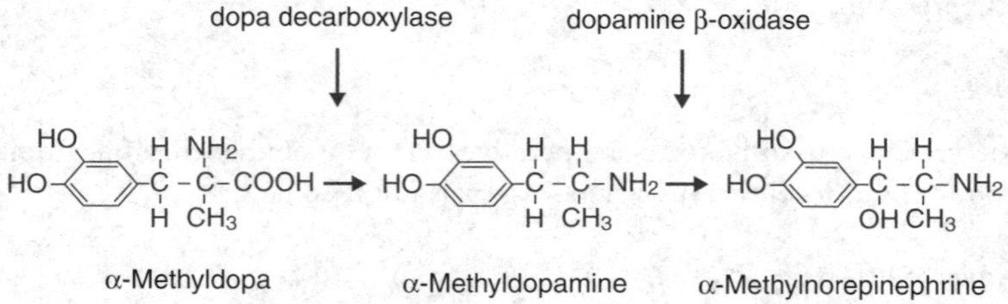

Figure 6–4 The metabolism of methyldopa in adrenergic neurons. a-Methylnorepinephrine replaces norepinephrine in neurosecretory vesicles.

B. Clonidine

Action

Clonidine stimulates α_2-receptors in the medulla oblongata to decrease sympathetic activity transmitted from the brain to the peripheral sympathetic nerves.

Clonidine reduces blood pressure by decreasing cardiac output. The decrease in cardiac output is due to a reduction in heart rate and dilation of the veins leading to a diminished venous return. Clonidine also dilates arterioles, but its ability to lower blood pressure correlates better with a decreased cardiac output than a reduced peripheral resistance.

Uses

Clonidine is used primarily to treat mild to moderate hypertension that has not responded to a diuretic and is usually administered along with a diuretic.

Adverse Effects

Sedation, dry mouth, edema, weight gain, and dizziness. Rebound hypertension if suddenly withdrawn.

ADRENERGIC RECEPTOR BLOCKERS

1. α-Blockers

A. Nonselective α-Blockers (Phentolamine, Tolazoline)

Actions

Phentolamine and tolazoline produce an equilibrium-competitive inhibition of the actions of catecholamines (epinephrine, norepinephrine, and dopamine) on α_1- and α_2-receptors. Because these drugs block α_2-adrenergic receptors, they increase the release of norepinephrine from sympathetic nerves. This leads to tachycardia as a result of increased β_1-adrenergic receptor stimulation.

Uses

These drugs have limited clinical use because of the tachycardia and other adverse effects they produce. Phentolamine is used to control blood pressure during surgery for pheochromocytoma and in the short-term control of hypertension in patients with a pheochromocytoma.

Adverse Effects

Postural hypotension, tachycardia, nasal congestion, nausea, vomiting, diarrhea.

B. Selective α_1-Adrenergic Blockers (Prazosin, Terazosin, Doxazosin)

Actions

These drugs produce a selective equilibrium-competitive block of α_1-adrenergic receptors. In normal clinical doses they do not block α_2-receptors. Because they block α_1-receptors, these drugs dilate both arterioles and veins, leading to a reduction in peripheral resistance and venous return.

Uses

These drugs are primarily used to treat hypertension.

They may also be used to treat benign prostatic hyperplasia. α_1-Adrenergic receptors in the trigone muscle of the bladder and urethra contribute to the resistance of urine outflow. Selective α_1-adrenergic receptor blockers reduce this resistance in some patients with impaired bladder emptying that has been caused by prostatic obstruction. They are effective in benign prostatic hyperplasia because they relax smooth muscle in the bladder neck, prostate capsules, and prostatic urethra.

Adverse Effects

Reflex tachycardia, postural hypotension, nasal congestion, gastrointestinal hypermotility, inhibition of ejaculation, fluid retention, weakness, dizziness, headache, lethargy.

2. β-Blockers

Table 6–1 reviews the distribution of β-receptors in the body and Table 6–2 compares the actions of the three groups of β-blockers.

A. Nonselective β-Adrenergic Blockers (Propranolol, Nadolol, Timolol)

Actions

Nonselective β-blockers competitively block both β_1- and β_2-adrenergic receptors. As a result of these actions, nonselective β-blockers
- decrease heart rate,
- decrease atrioventricular (AV) conduction,

Table 6–1

Distribution of Beta Receptors

Organ	Receptor Type	Effects of Stimulation
Heart	Beta$_1$ Beta$_1$ Beta$_1$	Increase in heart rate Increase in cardiac contractility Acceleration of AV conduction
Bronchioles	Beta$_2$	Dilation
Arterioles	Beta$_2$	Dilation
Kidney	Beta$_1$	Release of renin
Metabolic	Beta$_2$ Beta$_1$	Increase in blood sugar Increase in free fatty acids

AV = atrioventricular.

- decrease myocardial contractility and cardiac output,
- decrease blood pressure,
- decrease renin release,
- decrease FEV$_1$ in asthmatic patients,
- increase peripheral resistance, and
- decrease blood sugar.

Uses

Nonselective β-blockers are used to
- treat essential hypertension,
- manage angina pectoris,
- treat supraventricular arrhythmias,
- prevent migraine headaches (propranolol — mechanism of action unclear),
- decrease the peripheral manifestations of hyperthyroidism,
- reduce essential tremor (propranolol),
- control blood pressure prior to surgery in patients with pheochromocytoma (used in combination with a nonselective α-blocker), and
- reduce intraocular pressure in glaucoma (timolol instilled in the eye reduces the formation of aqueous humor — mechanism of action unclear).

Adverse Effects

Bronchoconstriction in asthmatics, increase in the hypoglycemic effects of insulin, asystole, AV block, bradycardia, heart failure, nausea, vomiting, constipation, diarrhea, CNS depression, sleep disturbances, allergic reactions.

Table 6–2
Differences Between Groups of Beta Blockers

	Non-Selective β-Blockers (Propranolol, Nadolol, Timolol)	Cardioselective β-Blockers (Acebutolol, Atenolol, Betaxolol, Esmolol, Metoprolol)	β-Blockers with ISA: Partial Agonist β-Blockers (Acebutolol, Oxprenolol, Pindolol)
Heart Rate and Force of Contraction (β_1)	Decrease both rate and force of contraction	Decrease both rate and force of contraction	Decrease both rate and force of contraction. Produce less of a fall in resting heart rate than non-selective or cardioselective β-blockers because of their ISA
Peripheral Resistance (β_2)	Increase, due to the fact that α_1-receptors can act unopposed by β_2-stimulation	Little change because β_2-receptors are not blocked	May be a slight decrease because of partial β_2-agonist properties
Renin Release (β_1)	Decrease release.	Decease release.	Decrease release
Bronchioles (β_2)	Bronchoconstriction in asthmatics.	Produce less bronchoconstriction than non-selective β-blockers but still not recommended in asthmatics	Reduce capacity of asthmatics to dilate bronchioles
Glucose Metabolism (β_2)	Prevent epinephrine from increasing blood sugar. As a result, insulin produces a greater and more prolonged fall in blood sugar. Use with caution in diabetics	Little effect.	Reduce response to epinephrine because partial agonist activity is not as potent as endogenously-released epinephrine

ISA = intrinsic sympathomimetic activity.

B. Cardioselective β-Adrenergic Blockers (Acebutolol, Atenolol, Betaxolol, Esmolol, Metoprolol)

Actions

Cardioselective β-blockers primarily block β_1-receptors. Because they do not block β_2-receptors, these drugs are less likely to

- prevent adrenergic dilation of the bronchioles,
- increase peripheral resistance, and
- potentiate the hypoglycemic actions of insulin.

Uses

Cardioselective β-blockers are used to

- treat essential hypertension,
- prevent attacks of angina pectoris,
- control ventricular arrhythmias in emergencies (esmolol),
- reduce intraocular pressure in glaucoma (betaxolol instilled in the eye reduces the formation of aqueous humor—mechanism of action is unclear).

Adverse Effects

As for non-selective β-adrenergic blockers, except they produce less bronchoconstriction, less effect on peripheral resistance, and less interaction with insulin.

C. β-Adrenergic Blockers with Intrinsic Sympathetic Activity (ISA): Partial Agonist β-Blockers (Acebutolol, Oxprenolol, Pindolol)

Actions

In contrast to the nonselective and cardioselective β-blockers, which attach to β-receptors and block them, β-blockers with ISA have affinity for β-receptors and, once attached, stimulate the receptors. However, because they have less intrinsic sympathetic activity than either epinephrine or norepinephrine, the degree of β-stimulation is reduced when acebutolol, oxprenolol, or pindolol occupies the receptor in place of the normal mediators, epinephrine and norepinephrine. These drugs are sometimes called **partial agonists**, a term that reflects their limited ability to stimulate adrenergic β-receptors.

Acebutolol is listed under both cardioselective β-blockers and β-blockers with ISA because this drug is a partial agonist that affects only β_1-receptors.

β-Blockers with ISA produce the same effects as nonselective β-blockers, except they

- do not decrease resting heart rate to the same degree as nonselective β-blockers,
- have less effect than nonselective β-blockers on the bronchioles, and
- produce a small decrease in peripheral resistance.

Uses

β-Adrenergic blockers with ISA are used to

- treat essential hypertension, and
- prevent attacks of angina pectoris.

Adverse Effects

As for non-selective β-blockers, except that they produce less bronchoconstriction and bradycardia.

3. α_1- and β-Blockers (Labetolol)

Action

Labetalol produces an equilibrium-competitive antagonism of α_1- and β-receptors. It is 3 to 7 times more potent as a non-selective β-blocker than an α_1-blocker. Labetalol is most appropriately thought of as a β-blocker with some α_1-blocking properties.

Labetalol's most important actions are exerted on the cardiovascular system:

- Labetalol combines the features of β- and α_1-blockade. When administered acutely, labetalol decreases peripheral vascular resistance (due to α_1-blockade and direct vascular effects), without an increase in cardiac rate and output (due to the β-blockade, which prevents the reflex increase in heart rate that is normally seen following a decrease in peripheral resistance).

- With prolonged therapy, the effects of β-blockade become more pronounced and labetalol decreases the heart rate. Generally, however, the decrease in heart rate is less pronounced than that seen after the administration of a β-blocker, such as propranolol. Prolonged treatment with labetalol also reduces vascular resistance and blood pressure.

Uses

Labetalol is used for

- the chronic treatment of essential hypertension, and
- the preoperative management of patients with a pheochromocytoma.

Adverse Effects

Postural hypotension, gastrointestinal distress, tiredness, sexual dysfunction, and a "tingling" of the scalp due to α_1-blockade.

Bronchospasm and congestive heart failure due to β-blockade.

These latter effects occur with a lower frequency than those associated with α_1-receptors.

7

Neuromuscular Blocking Drugs

COMPETITIVE BLOCKERS (NONDEPOLARIZING BLOCKERS) (TUBOCURARINE, ATRACURIUM, DOXACURIUM, GALLAMINE, METOCURINE, MIVACURIUM, PANCURONIUM, PIPERCURONIUM, ROCURONIUM, VECURONIUM)

Actions

These drugs competitively block nicotinic receptors on skeletal muscle, preventing acetylcholine, released from somatic nerves, from stimulating these receptors.

Tubocurarine also releases histamine, resulting in bronchospasm, hypotension, and excessive bronchial and salivary secretion.

Tubocurarine also releases heparin and this results in decreased blood coagulability.

The actions of these drugs can be terminated by administering a cholinesterase inhibitor, such as neostigmine. The resulting increased concentration of acetylcholine will overcome the competitive block of the nondepolarizing blocker.

Uses

Tubocurarine and the other competitive neuromuscular blockers are used as adjuvant drugs in surgical anesthesia. Neuromuscular blockers relax skeletal muscles and reduce the concentration of anesthetic required, thereby decreasing the risk of cardiovascular and respiratory depression. They are also used to prevent dislocations and fractures associated with electroconvulsive therapy and to control muscle spasms in tetanus.

Adverse Effects

Prolonged apnea. Because it releases histamine, tubocurarine can produce allergic responses, bronchospasm, excessive bronchial and salivary secretion, and hypotension.

DEPOLARIZING BLOCKERS (SUCCINYLCHOLINE)

Actions

Succinylcholine binds to acetylcholine nicotinic receptors on skeletal muscle to cause opening of ion channels, Na^+ influx, and depolarization of the muscle cell end-plate membrane in the same manner as acetylcholine. However, succinylcholine has a longer duration of action than acetylcholine because it is metabolized more slowly. As a result of the relatively slow metabolism of succinylcholine, the end-plate membrane remains **depolarized** with the ion channels remaining open. Neuromuscular blockade during depolarization is called **phase I block**.

In the continued presence of succinylcholine, depolarization may decrease so that Na^+-channel inactivation is reduced or reversed and muscle excitability is restored. Despite this change, the neuromuscular block continues. This condition is described as **phase II block**. The mechanism for **phase II block** is not understood.

Succinylcholine is metabolized by pseudocholinesterase. In patients with atypical pseudocholinesterase, succinylcholine is not metabolized rapidly and the drug has a prolonged duration of action.

Uses

Succinylcholine is used

- as an adjunct to anesthesia, to induce skeletal muscle relaxation, and
- to reduce the intensity of muscle contractions due to pharmacologically or electrically induced convulsions.

Adverse Effects

Profound and prolonged muscle relaxation in patients with atypical pseudocholinesterase, respiratory depression, bradycardia, tachycardia, hypertension, hypotension, cardiac arrest, and arrhythmias.

Part 3 Cardiovascular and
Renal Pharmacology

8

Drugs for the Treatment of Congestive Heart Failure

CONGESTIVE HEART FAILURE (CHF)

Heart Failure

Occurs following myocardial damage when the heart fails to pump enough blood to meet the needs of the tissues.

Edema Formation (Figure 8–1)

Congestion, dyspnea, and edema result from a complex series of events that occur when cardiac contractility falls.

Compensating Mechanisms in Heart Failure (Figure 8–2)

1. Increased heart size
2. Increased release of renin, with resulting increase in the synthesis of angiotensin II and aldosterone
   As a result:
   • angiotensin II constricts resistance vessels
   • aldosterone promotes salt and water retention
3. Increased sympathetic vasoconstriction

Consequences of Compensating Mechanisms

1. Increased systemic vascular resistance (afterload)
2. Increased blood volume
3. Increased venoconstriction (preload)

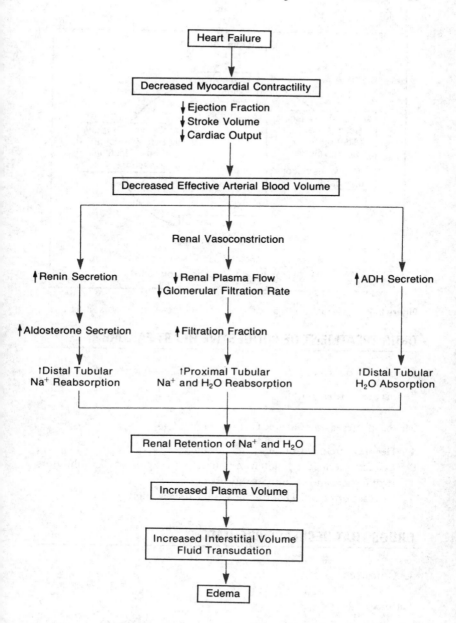

Figure 8–1 Schematic diagram of the renal causes of edema formation in heart failure. (After Young JB, Robert R. Heart failure. In: Dirks JH, Sutton RAL eds. Diuretics, physiology, pharmacology and clinical use. Philadelphia: W.B. Saunders, 1986:155.)

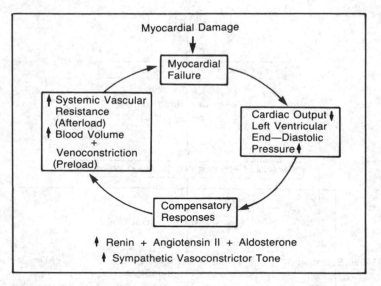

Figure 8–2 Compensating mechanisms in heart failure. (After Bristol-Myers Squibb.)

DRUG TREATMENT OF CONGESTIVE HEART FAILURE

Purpose of Treatment

To increase cardiac output.

Means of Increasing Cardiac Output (Figure 8–3)

1. Decrease preload (diuretics and nitrates)
2. Reduce afterload [angiotensin converting enzyme (ACE) inhibitors, hydralazine, and sodium nitroprusside]
3. Increase myocardial contractility (inotropic agents)

DRUGS THAT DECREASE PRELOAD

1. Diuretics

Actions

The pharmacologic actions of diuretics are presented in detail in Chapter 13.

These drugs, which include the thiazides, chlorthalidone, and loop diuretics, increase sodium, chloride, and water excretion.

They decrease blood volume and lower cardiac filling pressure, thereby reducing both pulmonary congestion and peripheral edema.

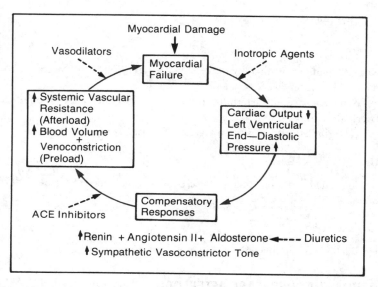

Figure 8–3 Use of diuretics, vasodilators and inotropic drugs to treat congestive heart failure. ACE= angiotensin converting enzyme. (Reproduced with permission of Bristol-Myers Squibb.)

Uses

Diuretics are first-line agents for all grades of cardiac failure when sinus rhythm is present.

They are usually sufficient to treat mild CHF.

For more severe CHF, diuretics are usually given with other drugs, such as a vasodilator and/or digoxin.

When symptoms are mild, less potent diuretics, such as the thiazides or chlorthalidone, may suffice.

In more severe cases, a loop diuretic, such as furosemide may be required.

Potassium loss is a common problem with diuretics. This effect can be reduced by combining these drugs with a potassium-sparing diuretic, such as triamterene, amiloride, or spironolactone, or by adding a potassium chloride preparation to the treatment regimen.

Adverse Effects

Hypovolemia, reduced renal perfusion, increased blood urea, hyponatremia, and hypokalemia. Mild to moderate hypokalemia can potentiate digoxin toxicity. Other adverse effects include hyperglycemia, hypercalcemia, magnesium depletion, and hyperlipidemia.

2. Nitrates

Actions

Nitrates dilate veins, thereby decreasing preload. This action accounts for their major beneficial effect in CHF.

Nitrates also dilate arterioles (precapillary resistance vessels) to reduce afterload.

Isosorbide dinitrate is the nitrate used most frequently.

Uses

May be added to diuretic therapy if a second drug is needed to further reduce preload.

Adverse Effects

Headache and hypotension are the most common adverse effects.

DRUGS THAT DECREASE AFTERLOAD

1. Angiotensin Converting Enzyme (ACE) Inhibitors (Captopril, Enalapril, Lisinopril)

Actions (Figures 8–4, 8–5, and 8–6)

By dilating precapillary resistance vessels (arterioles), ACE inhibitors reduce the systemic vascular resistance. In the face of a reduced systemic vascular

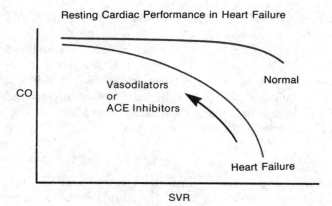

Figure 8–4 Diagrammatic representation of the consequences of reducing the systemic vascular resistance (SVR) on the cardiac output (CO) of the normal heart and the heart in failure. (After Bristol-Myers Squibb.)

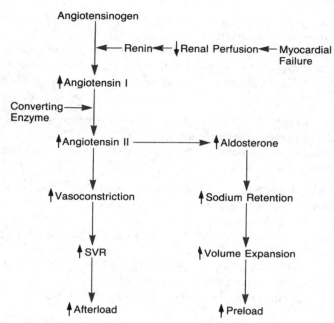

Figure 8–5 Contribution of the renin-angiotensin-aldosterone system to congestive heart failure. SVR = systemic vascular resistance. (After Bristol-Myers Squibb.)

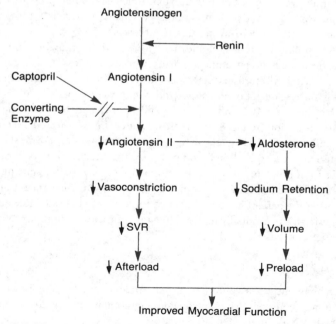

Figure 8–6 Effect of captopril on the renin-angiotensin-aldosterone system in congestive heart failure. SVR = systemic vascular resistance. (After Bristol-Myers Squibb.)

resistance, afterload falls and the heart in failure is more able to pump blood; therefore, cardiac output increases.

Myocardial failure causes an increase in renin secretion by the kidneys. Renin is converted to angiotensin I, which is, in turn, converted to angiotensin II by the angiotensin converting enzyme. Angiotensin II has two major effects:

- It constricts blood vessels. Constricting arterioles increases systemic vascular resistance and afterload.
- It increases aldosterone secretion, giving rise to sodium retention, volume expansion, and an increase in preload.

ACE inhibitors block the conversion of angiotensin I to angiotensin II, thereby dilating arterioles and reducing afterload.

By lowering angiotensin II and reducing venoconstriction, ACE inhibitors also decrease both right- and left-sided filling pressures (reduced preload).

By decreasing aldosterone secretion, ACE inhibitors reduce blood volume, further contributing to a decrease in preload.

The consequences of these actions lead to an improvement in CHF.

Uses

ACE inhibitors are effective in treating chronic CHF. Blood pressure often falls initially, but if the patient is not hypertensive, it usually returns to a value not significantly below pretreatment levels.

ACE inhibitors are useful additions to diuretic therapy because they reduce both the hyponatremia and urinary potassium loss.

If an ACE inhibitor is used, the patient should not receive a potassium-sparing diuretic or potassium supplement to prevent hyperkalemia.

The effects of ACE inhibitors depend on the patient's salt balance. Sodium depletion activates the renin-angiotensin system and increases ACE inhibitor activity. Patients on high-dose diuretic therapy are most likely to experience a severe fall in blood pressure after the first dose or doses of an ACE inhibitor. Diuretics are often stopped a few days before starting low doses of an ACE inhibitor to minimize the initial hypotensive effect of the drug. After the patient has demonstrated the ability to tolerate these doses, the physician can gradually increase the dose of the ACE inhibitor to meet the patient's needs.

Adverse Effects

Severe hypotension in volume depleted patients, modest deterioration in renal function, proteinuria, neutropenia, alteration in taste (with captopril), skin rash, cough, angioedema.

2. Hydralazine

Actions

Hydralazine effectively dilates precapillary resistance vessels (arterioles), with minimal effect on the capacitance vessels (veins).

Its mechanism of action is not clear.

In heart failure, hydralazine reduces right and left ventricular afterload by reducing systemic and pulmonary vascular resistance. These actions result in an increase of forward stroke volume and a reduction in both ventricular systolic wall stress and regurgitant fraction in mitral insufficiency.

Because of the decrease in peripheral resistance, hydralazine can increase heart rate (HR), raise the release of renin, the synthesis of angiotensin II, and the secretion of aldosterone.

Hydralazine is inactivated by acetylation; therefore, slow acetylators should receive lower doses.

Uses

Hydralazine has minimal effect on venous capacitance and therefore is most effective when combined with venodilators, such as organic nitrates.

Hydralazine reduces renal vascular resistance and increases renal blood flow to a greater degree than most other vasodilators.

As a result of these actions, hydralazine may be the vasodilator of choice in heart failure patients with renal dysfunction who cannot tolerate an ACE inhibitor.

Adverse Effects

Headache, tachycardia, anorexia, dizziness, sweating.

3. Sodium Nitroprusside

Actions

Nitroprusside dilates both precapillary resistance and capacitance vessels, thereby decreasing both afterload and preload, respectively.

Nitroprusside is one of the most effective afterload-reducing drugs because of its effects on different vascular beds. Nitroprusside

- decreases peripheral vascular resistance,
- increases aortic wall compliance,
- improves ventricular-vascular coupling, as well as cardiac output, and
- dilates pulmonary arterioles and reduces right ventricular afterload.

This combination of preload- and afterload-reducing effects improves myocardial productivity by reducing wall stress, provided that blood pressure does not fall to the point of compromising diastolic coronary artery flow, or to the point of activating a marked reflex increase in sympathetic nervous system tone.

Uses

Nitroprusside is particularly effective in patients with congestive heart failure caused by mitral regurgitation or left-to-right shunts through a ventricular septal defect.

Adverse Effects

Flushing, headache, hypotension, nausea, vomiting, anorexia, muscle spasms, hypoxia, methemoglobinemia, increased blood levels of thiocyanate and cyanide.

DRUGS THAT INCREASE MYOCARDIAL CONTRACTILITY (INOTROPIC DRUGS)

1. Digoxin

A. Mechanical Actions

Increased Myocardial Contractility

Digoxin improves myocardial contractility by increasing the intensity of the interaction of actin and myosin filaments of the cardiac sarcomere. This increased intensity is caused by an increase in the free calcium concentration in the vicinity of the contractile proteins during systole. Digoxin:

- Inhibits membrane Na^+, K^+-ATPase transport function, causing accumulation of intracellular Na^+. Elevated intracellular Na^+ levels reduce calcium expulsion from the myocardial cell by the Na^+- Ca^{++} exchanger. The resulting rise in intracellular calcium in the vicinity of the contractile proteins during systole increases myocardial contractility
- Facilitates calcium entry into the myocardial cell through the voltage-gated calcium channels of the membrane
- Increases the release of calcium from intracellular storage sties on sarcoplasmic reticulum

Decreased Peripheral Resistance

Because of the improved performance of the heart, the need for increased sympathetic stimulation of the precapillary resistance vessels is eliminated.

As a result of a reduction in norepinephrine release, the vessels dilate and tissue perfusion improves.

Decreased Heart Rate and AV Conduction

Initially, prior to treatment, increased sympathetic stimulation increases HR. Once myocardial performance improves under the influence of digoxin, the need for increased sympathetic drive to the heart decreases. Normal vagal tone returns and heart rate and atrioventricular (AV) conduction decrease.

B. Electrical Actions (Figure 8–7, Table 8–1)

Increased Automaticity

Digoxin increases spontaneous diastolic depolarization (see phase 4 in Figure 8–7).

Decreased Conductivity

Digoxin decreases conductivity. This is reflected by a decrease in the rate of rise and amplitude of the action potential.

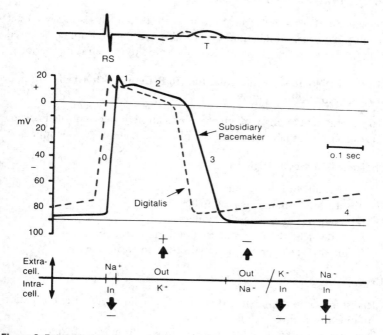

Figure 8–7 Effects of digoxin on subsidiary pacemaker activity. (After Mason DT, Zelis R, et al. Current concepts and treatment of digitalis toxicity. Am J Cadiol 1971;27:547.)

Table 8–1

Summary of the Direct and Vagal-Mediated Effects of Digoxin on Heart-Dominant Mechanisms

Area of Heart	Automaticity		Conductivity		Refractory Period	
	Direct	Vagal	Direct	Vagal	Direct	Vagal
SA Node	Increase	*Decrease*	Decrease	*Decrease*	Decrease	*Increase*
Atria			Decrease	*Increase*	Decrease	*Decrease*
AV Conductivity	Increase	*Decrease*	Decrease	*Decrease*	Decrease	*Increase*
Purkinje	*Increase*		Decrease		Decrease	

Dominant mechanisms in normal therapeutic doses are indicated in italics. AV = atrioventricular; SA = sinoatrial.

Decreased Refractory Period

Digoxin shortens the duration of the action potential (see phases 1, 2, and 3 in Figure 8–7) and thus decreases the refractory period.

The overall effect of digoxin on the heart is a balance between its direct actions (increased automoticity, decreased conductivity, and decreased refractory period) and the consequences of increased vagal activity (see Table 8–1).

Effects of Digoxin on Atrial Flutter

Digoxin often converts atrial flutter to atrial fibrillation. This is largely a result of increased vagal stimulation. On **atrial muscle,** acetylcholine, released from the vagus, increases conductivity and shortens the refractory period.

Effects of Digoxin On Ventricular Rate in Patients With Atrial Flutter or Atrial Fibrillation

Despite the fact that digoxin often converts atrial flutter to fibrillation, the ventricular rate usually slows because of the delay in AV conduction.

Pharmacokinetics of Digoxin

- Given orally or intravenously
- Absorption from tablets is 60 to 80%
- Eliminated primarily by the kidneys
- Half-life of 1.5 days in patients with normal renal function
- Reduce dosage in proportion to decrease in creatinine clearance

Uses

Clearest indication is in patients with cardiac failure and atrial fibrillation with uncontrolled ventricular response.

Its use in heart failure with normal sinus rhythm is controversial.

Adverse Effects

- Sinus bradycardia
- Paroxysmal or nonparoxysmal atrial tachycardia
- Conversion of atrial flutter to atrial fibrillation
- Increases automaticity in AV tissue, leading to junctional rhythms, including tachycardia
- Premature ventricular depolarizations (bigeminy, ventricular tachycardia, ventricular fibrillation)
- Complete heart block
- Anorexia, nausea, vomiting, abdominal discomfort, diarrhea
- CNS effects — headache, fatigue, malaise, drowsiness, blurred vision
- Conditions which increase digoxin's actions on the heart include hypokalemia, hypothyroidism, age, and myocardial infarction.

2. Amrinone

Actions

Amrinone inhibits phosphodiesterase, thereby increasing the uptake of Ca^{++} by myocardial cells.

This action may account for the ability of amrinone to increase myocardial contractility and dilate vascular smooth muscle.

Amrinone decreases both preload and afterload and reduces left and right ventricular filling pressures and pulmonary capillary wedge pressure.

It improves resting and exercise hemodynamics, increases left ventricular ejection fraction, and improves ventricular capacity.

Uses

Amrinone is used in patients with severe CHF not adequately controlled by digoxin, diuretics, antiarrhythmic drugs, or vasodilators.

It is also used in patients with refractory acute heart failure due to myocardial infarction.

Adverse Effects

Thrombocytopenia, fever, and nephrogenic diabetes insipidus.

3. Dobutamine and Dopamine

Refer to Chapter 5 for information on these drugs.

9

Drugs for the Treatment of Cardiac Arrhythmias

ETIOLOGY OF CARDIAC ARRHYTHMIAS

Cardiac Arrhythmias

Are caused by disorders of rate, rhythm, origin, or conduction within the heart.

Cardiac Tachyarrhythmias

Are the result of disorders of

- impulse formation,
- impulse conduction, or
- both.

DISORDERS OF IMPULSE FORMATION

- The heart has many cells that have the potential to act as pacemakers. These cells are referred to as **latent pacemakers** and are found in specialized conducting systems, such as the atrioventricular (AV) node, the AV bundle, and the Purkinje network in the ventricles. These cells have the property of **automaticity** because they can depolarize spontaneously.
- **Latent pacemakers** have the potential to act as ectopic **pacemakers.** Under normal circumstances, they do not function as pacemakers because the sinoatrial (SA) node depolarizes more rapidly and serves as the site for impulse formation. Once the SA node reaches its threshold, it sends an electrical wave throughout the heart, depolarizing all latent pacemakers before they have a chance to act as sites of impulse conduction.

- If the normal SA pacemaker node is damaged, or if the rate of conduction of impulses from the SA node is reduced, formerly latent pacemakers may become **ectopic pacemakers**.

DISORDERS OF IMPULSE CONDUCTION

- Disorders of impulse conduction are more often the cause of cardiac arrhythmias than disorders of impulse formation.
- AV blocks or bundle branch blocks cause arrhythmias.
- Re-entry (Figure 9–1) can cause paroxysmal tachycardias and ventricular tachycardias. If a localized area of the heart is damaged by a myocardial infarct, the transmission of impulses along a portion of a normal conducting system may be blocked in one direction. In Figure 9–1, impulse transmission is blocked unidirectionally along pathway *b*. As a result, the impulse that travels along *a* and *c* is allowed to come up *b* in a retrograde manner and re-enter *a* in the manner shown. This results in an extra heartbeat. If it happens at several sites, it can produce severe tachyarrhythmias leading to fibrillation.

PHARMACOLOGIC APPROACHES TO TREATING TACHYARRHYTHMIAS

Cardiac tachyarrhythmias may be treated by:

- reducing the rate at which ectopic pacemakers depolarize, or
- modifying the conduction defects that lead to re-entry. Re-entry mechanisms can be altered either by:
  - ◆ increasing the conductivity in the damaged tissue, or
  - ◆ further decreasing the conduction velocity, thereby converting a undirectional block to a bidirectional one. A bidirectional block is depicted in Figure 9–2.

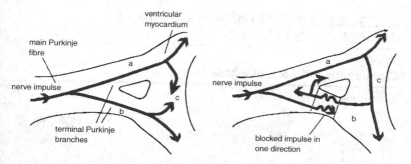

A. Impulse conduction with healthy myocardium   B. Impulse conduction impaired by myocardial infarct

Figure 9–1 The phenomenon of re-entry. (After Johnson GE, Osis M, Hannah KJ. Pharmacology in Nursing Practice. Toronto: W.B. Saunders, 1998.)

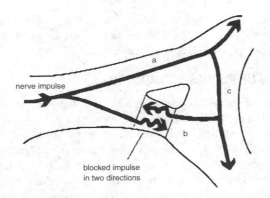

Figure 9–2 Bidirectional block. (After Johnson GE, Osis M, Hannah KJ. Pharmacology in Nursing Practice. Toronto: W.B. Saunders, 1998.)

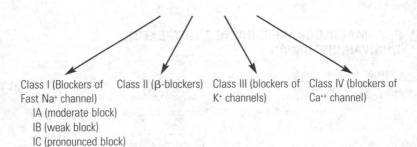

Class I (Blockers of   Class II (β-blockers)   Class III (blockers of   Class IV (blockers of
Fast Na⁺ channel)   K⁺ channels)   Ca⁺⁺ channel)
  IA (moderate block)
  IB (weak block)
  IC (pronounced block)

Figure 9–3 Classification of Antiarrhythmic Drugs

CLASSIFICATION OF ANTIARRHYTHMIC DRUGS (FIGURE 9–3 AND TABLE 9–1)

Table 9–1
Classification of Antiarrhythmic Drugs

Antiarrhythmic Class	Representative Drugs	Principal Pharmacologic Effects
Class IA	Quinidine Procainamide Disopyramide	**All Class I antiarrhythmic drugs** (Class IA, Class IB, and Class IC) reduce sodium entry at the time the cell membrane rapidly depolarizes (ie, they decrease the fast inward sodium current). As a result, Class I drugs decrease the rate of depolarization Continued

Table 9–1
Classification of Antiarrhythmic Drugs—Continued

Antiarrhythmic Class	Representative Drugs	Principal Pharmacologic Effects
		In their presence, cells require a greater (more negative) potential before they can propagate an impulse to adjacent cells (ie, they increase the threshold to impulse propagation). Class I drugs also increase the repolarization time, reduce conduction velocity, prolong the effective refractory period, and decrease automaticity. **Class IA** drugs depress automaticity, particularly at ectopic sites and slow conduction and increase the refractoriness of the atria, the His-Purkinje system, accessory pathways, and the ventricles. They have both direct and indirect (anticholinergic) actions (Table 9–2).
Class IB	Lidocaine Mexiletine Phenytoin Tocainide	**For properties of all Class I antiarrhythmic drugs see comments above. Class IB drugs depress automaticity and** reduce the duration of the refractory period in the His-Purkinje system and the ventricles. In therapeutic doses, they do not slow AV nodal or intraventricular conduction, except in diseased myocardium.
Class IC	Flecainide Moricizine Propafenone	**For properties of all Class I antiarrhythmic drugs see comments above. Flecainide and propafenone** slow conduction in the atria, AV node, ventricles, accessory pathways, and particularly in the His-Purkinje system. To a lesser extent, they also increase atrial and ventricular refractoriness and suppress sinus node automaticity. Moricizine does not readily fit into any of the subclasses of drugs that block sodium channels and has proven difficult to subclassify within the Class I antiarrhythmic agents. It reduces the fast inward sodium current of the action potential, prolongs atria to His (AH) and His to ventricle (HV) conduction times, and PR and QRS intervals.
Class II	Propranolol Metoprolol Nadolol	**Class II antiarrhythmic** drugs are competitive β-blockers. By blocking β$_1$ receptors, these drugs reduce cardiac

Continued

Table 9–1

Classification of Antiarrhythmic Drugs—Continued

Antiarrhythmic Class	Representative Drugs	Principal Pharmacologic Effects
	Acebutolol Atenolol Pindolol Timolol Sotalol Esmolol	output, diminish myocardial oxygen requirements, and prevent cardiac arrhythmias, particularly those caused by increased sympathetic activity (see Chapter 6). The cardiac effects of β_1-blockage include: • bradycardia • decreased contractility • increased AV conduction time • reduced automaticity
Class III	Amiodarone Bretylium Sotalol	**Class III antiarrhythmic drugs** inhibit potassium repolarization. **Amiodarone** increases refractoriness of the sinus node, the atria, the AV node, the ventricles, the His-Purkinje system, and the accessory pathways; depresses sinus node automaticity; and slows conduction in the atria, the AV node, the His-Purkinje system, and the ventricles. **Bretylium** has two actions — it directly modifies the electrical properties of the myocardium, and it initially increases norepinephrine release and subsequently depresses adrenergic neuronal transmission. The initial release of norepinephrine increases automaticity. Subsequently, bretylium increases the refractory period of the His-Purkinje system and ventricles without slowing conduction or depressing automaticity. **Sotalol** is both a noncardioselective β-blocker and a drug with class III antiarrhythmic properties that prolongs atrial and ventricular refractoriness.
Class IV	Verapamil Diltiazem	**Class IV antiarrhythmic drugs** are calcium channel blockers, which selectively inhibit the slow-channel calcium ion transport into cardiac tissue. The pacemakers of the SA node and the cells in the proximal region of the AV node are depolarized primarily by the calcium current. Blocking the calcium channel has the effect of depressing AV conduction, thereby reducing the ability of the AV node to conduct supraventricular impulses to the ventricle. The most important electrocardiogram (ECG) change is a prolongation of the PR interval.

CLASS IA ANTIARRHYTHMIC DRUGS
(QUINIDINE, PROCAINAMIDE, DISOPYRAMIDE)

Actions

Quinidine, procainamide, and disopyramide reduce the maximum rate of depolarization. They

- increase the threshold for excitation,
- depress conduction velocity, and
- prolong the effective refractory period

in the atrial, His-bundle, and ventricular conducting systems.

These drugs also exert a direct anticholinergic (atropine-like) effect on the muscarinic receptors of the heart (see Chapter 4). A summary of the effects of these drugs is presented in Table 9–2.

Uses and Adverse Effects

1. Quinidine

Used to treat both atrial and ventricular arrhythmias.

Has been used to maintain sinus rhythm after cardioversion in supraventricular arrhythmias.

Table 9–2
Electrophysiologic Actions of Quinidine, Procainamide and Disopyramide at Therapeutic Plasma Concentrations

Tissue	Direct Action	Indirect AC* Action	Net Effect
Sinus node depolarization	Decrease	Increase	No change
Atrial tissue			
Conduction velocity	Decrease	Decrease	Decrease
Effective refractory period	Increase	Increase	Increase
AV node			
Automaticity	Decrease	Increase	Increase/decrease[†]
Conduction velocity	Decrease	Increase	Increase/decrease[†]
Effective refractory period	Increase	Decrease	Decrease/increase[†]
His-Purkinje system – ventricular muscle			
Automaticity	Decrease	—	Decrease
Conduction velocity	Decrease	—	Decrease
Effective refractory period	Increase	—	Increase

(After Black SC, Lucchesi BR. Antiarrhythmic Drugs. In: Craig CR, Stitzel RE, eds. Modern pharmacology. Boston: Little, Brown, 1994:285.)
*Anticholinergic
[†]Dose-dependent effect (low dose/high dose)

Often used with digoxin to treat atrial fibrillation. Because quinidine has an atropinic action, it increases AV conduction. Digoxin, on the other hand, decreases AV conduction. By combining the two drugs, the physician can slow the atria with quinidine and reduce AV conduction with digoxin.

Quinidine's toxicities are usually dose related.

At plasma concentrations above 8 µg/mL, the direct depressant effects on AV conduction appear and the QRS complex widens. As the concentration of drug rises, SA block or arrest, high-grade AV block, ventricular arrhythmias, or asystole may occur.

The other adverse effects of quinidine include diarrhea, nausea and vomiting, headache, vertigo, palpitations, tinnitus and visual disturbances.

GI symptoms are the most common. They occur even when the drug concentrations in the plasma are low.

2. Procainamide

Possesses little atropinic action.

Has essentially the same therapeutic effects and clinical indications as quinidine.

Used to treat atrial fibrillation and paroxysmal supraventricular tachycardia.

Should not be administered to patients with complete AV heart block and is contraindicated in cases of second-degree and third-degree AV block unless an electric pacemaker is operative.

May cause anorexia, nausea, vomiting, granulocytopenia, and a reversible lupus erythematosus-like syndrome.

Both procainamide, and its active metabolite N-acetylprocainamide are eliminated by the kidneys and will accumulate in patients with renal impairment unless lower doses are given. Unless the serum concentrations of procainamide can be measured, it is better not to use the drug in end-stage renal failure.

3. Disopyramide

Has actions and uses similar to those of quinidine.

Eliminated by both hepatic metabolism and renal excretion, and therefore, dosage should be reduced in patients with liver or kidney impairment.

Contraindicated in the presence of shock, renal failure, severe intraventricular conduction defects, pre-existing second- and third-degree AV block (if no pacemaker is present), and known hypersensitivity to the drug.

Should not be used in the presence of uncompensated or inadequately compensated congestive heart failure because it can worsen the condition.

Severe hypotension occurring after disopyramide has been observed, usually in patients with primary myocardial disease (cardiomyopathy), and in patients with inadequately compensated CHF or advanced myocardial disease with low output states.

Other adverse effects include heart block, ventricular fibrillation, and tachyarrhythmias.

Its anticholinergic effects are often marked, and the drug is contraindicated in most patients with glaucoma and in those with urinary retention.

CLASS IB ANTIARRHYTHMIC DRUGS (LIDOCAINE, MEXILETINE, PHENYTOIN, TOCAINIDE)

Actions

See Table 9–1.

Uses and Adverse Effects

1. Lidocaine

Used for the immediate control of ventricular premature extrasystoles and ventricular tachycardia.

Also used for ventricular arrhythmias secondary to cardiac surgery, cardiac catheterization, acute myocardial infarction, and electrical conversion.

Major toxicities involve the CNS and the cardiovascular system (CVS). Patients may experience drowsiness, paresthesias, muscle twitching, convulsion, coma, respiratory depression, and depressed myocardial contractility.

Rapidly metabolized and patients with hepatic insufficiency and those over 70 age should, as a rule, receive ½ to ⅔ the usual loading dose and lower than normal maintenance doses.

2. Mexiletine

Used to treat or prevent ventricular ectopy and tachycardia and to suppress ventricular arrhythmias in survivors of acute myocardial infarction following therapy with lidocaine.

CVS toxicities include sinus bradycardia or tachycardia, atrial fibrillation, hypotension, dyspnea, ventricular tachyarrhythmias, including torsades de pointes.

Contraindicated in the presence of second- or third-degree AV block in the absence of a pacemaker, and in cardiogenic shock.

Use with caution in patients with hypotension or CHF because of its potential for depression of myocardial contractility.

Noncardiac adverse reactions include nausea, vomiting, malaise, dizziness, tremor, diplopia, paresthesias, confusion, and ataxia.

3. Phenytoin

Depresses spontaneous atrial and ventricular automaticity without altering intraventricular conduction.

May also increase conduction through damaged Purkinje fibers.

Used mainly to reverse digitalis-induced arrhythmias.

Adverse effects include fatigue, dizziness, ataxia, nausea, vomiting, pruritus, and rashes.

If given rapidly by intravenous (IV), it can slow the heart rate, depress the myocardium, produce hypotension, reduce AV conduction, and, very occasionally, cause cardiac arrest.

Contraindicated in sinus bradycardia, SA block, second- and third-degree AV block, and Adams-Stokes syndrome.

4. Tocainide

Indicated only for the treatment of symptomatic ventricular arrhythmias in patients not responding to other therapy, or when other therapy was not tolerated.

Use with caution in patients with heart failure or with minimal cardiac reserve because of the potential for aggravating the degree of heart failure.

Nausea and tremor are the most common adverse effects. Other adverse effects include dizziness, lightheadedness, confusion, anxiety, paresthesias, hypotension, bradycardia, palpitations, chest pain, conduction disturbances, and left ventricular failure. There are also reports of hematologic disorders, including leukopenia, agranulocytosis, bone marrow depression, hypoplastic anemia, and thrombocytopenia.

CLASS IC ANTIARRHYTHMIC DRUGS (FLECAINIDE, MORICIZINE, PROPAFENONE)

Actions

See Table 9–1.

Uses and Adverse Effects

1. Flecainide

Indicated for the treatment of documented ventricular arrhythmias, such as sustained ventricular tachycardia, that are judged life-threatening.

Most serious adverse reactions are new or exacerbated ventricular arrhythmias and new or worsened CHF.

Other adverse effects include blurred vision, dizziness, headache, nausea, fatigue, nervousness, tremor, and paresthesias.

2. Moricizine

In patients with impaired left ventricular function, moricizine has minimal effects on measurements of cardiac performance, such as cardiac index, stroke volume index, pulmonary capillary wedge pressure, and systemic or pulmonary vascular resistance or ejection fraction, either at rest or during exercise.

Used to suppress life-threatening ventricular arrhythmias.

CVS adverse effects include worsening of arrhythmias, conduction disturbances, and heart failure. Nausea and vomiting can also occur.

3. Propafenone

Used for suppression of the following ventricular arrhythmias when they occur singly or in combination: episodes of ventricular tachycardia; premature (ectopic) ventricular contractions, such as premature ventricular beats of unifocal or multifocal origin; couplets; and R on T phenomenon, when of sufficient severity to require treatment.

Adverse effects include worsening of CHF, AV and intraventricular conduction disturbances, ventricular arrhythmias, nausea, diarrhea, constipation, paresthesias, and taste disturbances.

CLASS II ANTIARRHYTHMIC DRUGS (BETA BLOCKERS)

Actions

See Table 9–1.

Uses and Adverse Effeccts

Beta blockers are best suited for catecholamine-induced arrhythmias.
   Beta blockers can be used to treat:

- Sinus tachycardia. First treat the underlying cause (eg, hyperpyrexia, hypovolemia, etc)
- Atrial fibrillation. Sinus rhythm is unlikely to be restored; however, the beta blockade of the AV node will decrease the ventricular response to the atrial tachyarrhythmia.
- Atrial flutter or tachycardia. Beta blockers will reduce the ventricular rate by inhibiting adrenergically mediated transmission through the AV node.
- Premature ventricular complexes. Effective in mitral valve prolapse, hypertrophic cardiomyopathy, digitalis-related ectopic activity, as well as ventricular complexes associated with exercise or induced by ischemia.
- Ventricular tachycardia. Most effective against arrhythmias associated with digitalis toxicity and exercise, particularly if the latter is related to ischemia.
- Ventricular fibrillation. Postmyocardial infarct patients show increased survival if treated with a β-blocker. The beneficial effect may be related to the decrease in heart rate and the anti-ischemic benefits from blocking the β-receptors.

For adverse effects, refer to Chapter 6.

CLASS III ANTIARRHYTHMIC DRUGS (AMIODARONE, BRETYLIUM, SOTALOL)

Actions

See Table 9–1.

Uses and Adverse Effects

The importance of class III antiarrhythmic drugs is their effectiveness in cases of intractable ventricular tachycardia and in reducing the likelihood of developing ventricular fibrillation.

Class III drugs may prolong the action-potential duration sufficiently to induce arrhythmias. This effect may relate to the ability of these drugs to sufficiently reduce potassium ion conductance to lead to a marked prolongation in repolarization.

1. **Amiodarone**

The prominent effect seen after acute IV administration of amiodarone is slow conduction and prolonged refractoriness of the AV node.

Amiodarone may also have a marked negative inotropic effect following acute IV administration.

Because of its toxicities, amiodarone is only indicated for the treatment of patients with life-threatening cardiac arrhythmias (eg, ventricular tachycardia and ventricular fibrillation) that are refractory to other treatments.

Amiodarone is contraindicated in severe sinus node dysfunctions, sinus bradycardia, and second- and third-degree AV block. It is also contraindicated in patients with episodes of bradycardia sufficient to cause syncope, unless used in conjunction with a pacemaker.

Amiodarone can be a most toxic drug. The most serious and potentially life-threatening adverse effects associated with its use are pulmonary fibrosis, aggravation of arrhythmias, and cirrhotic hepatitis.

Its effects on the CVS include myocardial depression, hypotension, SA block, AV block, ventricular arrhythmias, fatal CHF, cardiogenic shock, and cardiac arrest.

Other effects include headache, weakness, myalgia, tremor, ataxia, paresthesias, depression, insomnia, nightmares, and hallucinations.

2. **Bretylium**

Bretylium suppresses ventricular fibrillation and ventricular arrhythmias. As a result, it may be of value as a last resort in life-threatening ventricular arrhythmias, principally ventricular tachycardia and fibrillation, which are resistant to conventional antiarrhythmic drug therapy.

The major adverse effects of bretylium relate to its modification of adrenergic function. The catecholamines released shortly after its injection increase blood pressure and heart rate. This may be followed by the consequences of a subsequent sympathetic block (peripheral vasodilatation and profound, long-lasting hypotension).

The initial release of catecholamines may also cause anxiety, excitement, flushing, substernal pressure sensation, headache, and angina pectoris.

Rapid IV administration may initiate nausea and vomiting.

3. Sotalol

Sotalol is approved for the treatment of documented life-threatening ventricular arrhythmias, such as sustained ventricular tachycardia.

It may also be used for the treatment of patients with symptomatic ventricular arrhythmias.

Sotalol is contraindicated in patients with bronchial asthma, allergic rhinitis, severe sinus node dysfunction, sinus bradycardia, second- and third-degree AV block (unless a functioning pacemaker is present), and congenital or acquired long QT syndrome. The drug is also contraindicated in cardiogenic shock, severe or uncontrolled CHF, hypokalemia and anesthesia with agents that produce myocardial depression.

Adverse effects include those attributed to both beta blockade and proarrhythmic actions. The proarrhythmic effects of the drug may lead to ventricular fibrillation. For details on the adverse effects related to beta blockade, refer to Chapter 6.

CLASS IV ANTIARRHYTHMIC DRUGS (VERAPAMIL AND DILTIAZEM)

Actions

See Table 9–1.

Uses and Adverse Effects

1. Verapamil

IV administered verapamil can be used to treat paroxysmal supraventricular tachycardia (eg, atrial fibrillation or atrial flutter of recent onset with rapid ventricular response).

Oral verapamil is indicated for the treatment of atrial fibrillation or flutter with rapid ventricular response not otherwise controlled with digoxin.

Oral verapamil is also indicated as follow-up treatment to injectable verapamil in paroxysmal supraventricular tachycardia.

Because of its potent AV nodal depressant activity, verapamil should be used with caution, or not at all, in patients with AV nodal dysfunction, including those taking digitalis.

Contraindications to the use of verapamil also include acute myocardial infarction, severe congestive heart failure (unless secondary to a supraventricular tachycardia amenable to verapamil therapy), cardiogenic shock or severe hypotension, second- or third-degree AV block, sick sinus syndrome (except in patients with a functioning artificial ventricular pacemaker), and marked bradycardia.

The most common adverse effect following IV administration is a transient and mild fall in blood pressure.

Oral verapamil almost invariably causes constipation. Nausea, vomiting, lightheadedness, headache, flushing, nervousness, rashes and pruritus may also occur following oral treatment.

2. Diltiazem

The antiarrhythmic actions and uses of diltiazem are similar to those of verapamil.

Injectable diltiazem is indicated for the temporary control of rapid ventricular rate during atrial flutter or atrial fibrillation.

The contraindications to the use of diltiazem and the adverse effects of the drug are presented in Chapter 10.

MISCELLANEOUS ANTIARRHYTHMIC DRUGS

1. Digoxin

Actions

The actions of digoxin were presented in Chapter 8 (see Table 8–1 and Figure 8–7).

Lengthens the AV nodal conduction time and functional refractory period.

Slows the sinus rate when ventricular function is impaired because it increases cardiac output, leading to a reduction in sympathetic stimulation.

Uses and Adverse Effects

Slows the ventricular response in patients with atrial fibrillation or flutter. Because digoxin slows conduction over the AV node and increases the refractory period of the AV node, fewer impulses originating in the atria are able to invade the ventricular myocardium over the AV nodal pathway. Thus, despite the continued presence of a supraventricular arrhythmia, the ventricular rate will decrease, thereby improving cardiac hemodynamics.

Also used to treat AV nodal re-entrant tachycardia, and arrhythmias associated with congestive heart failure.

The adverse effects of digoxin were presented in Chapter 8.

2. Adenosine

Actions

The electrophysiologic actions of adenosine on the AV node resemble those of acetylcholine. Adenosine increases the effective refractory period and depresses conductivity.

When injected by IV, adenosine slows AV nodal conduction and can interrupt the re-entry pathways through the AV node.

Uses and Adverse Effects

Adenosine is indicated for the conversion of paroxysmal supraventricular tachycardia (PSVT) to normal sinus rhythm, including PSVT with Wolff-Parkinson-White syndrome.

Symptomatic adverse effects are common and include transient nausea, metallic taste, dyspnea, chest pain, ventricular ectopy, headache, and flushing.

10

Antianginal Drugs

Angina Pectoris:

- A syndrome of paroxysmal left-sided chest pain
- Produced when the oxygen requirements of the heart exceed the oxygen supply
- One of the most prominent and well-known symptoms of regional myocardial ischemia
- Caused most frequently by coronary artery disease

ANGINA CAUSED BY DISEASES OF CORONARY ARTERIES MAY BE DIVIDED INTO STABLE ANGINA AND VARIANT ANGINA

Stable Angina

Also called typical, classic, or exertional angina. Caused by a reduction of blood flow to a particular area of the heart as a result of atherosclerosis. Brought on by conditions that increase myocardial oxygen consumption, such as physical exertion, emotional stress, exposure to cold, or eating large meals.

Variant Angina

Also called vasospastic angina. Results from a coronary artery spasm. Develops typically at rest rather than during physical exertion; it frequently follows a diurnal rhythm, often occurring in the early morning. Not associated with an increased cardiac demand for oxygen, rather, the cause appears to be a spasm of one or more of the coronary arteries.

Both spasm and atheroma may be present in varying degrees

Objectives of Drug Treatment

1. To stop an existing attack or prevent a new one from occurring
2. To increase the exercise capacity of the patient

Means By Which These Objectives Can Be Reached

1. Increase the oxygen supply to the ischemic area(s) of the heart
2. Decrease the oxygen requirements of the heart muscle

For Stable Angina

The cause of the problem is a reduction in blood flow to an atherosclerotic area of the heart because hardened vessels cannot dilate. It is easier to decrease the myocardial oxygen requirements in stable angina than to increase the oxygen supply to the heart.

For Variant Angina

The blood vessels are not atherosclerotic in variant angina and, therefore, are able to dilate if treated with vasodilators. Thus, both nitrates and calcium channel blockers

- prevent the arteriole from going into spasm, and
- relax the arteriole that is in spasm.

Mechanisms of Action of Antianginal Drugs (Figure 10–1)

1. Reduce the heart rate (beta blockers)
2. Reduce preload (nitrates)

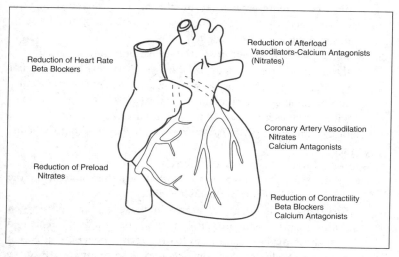

Figure 10–1 Mechanisms of action of anti-anginal drugs. (After Maclean D, Feely J. Calcium antagonists, nitrates and new anti-anginal drugs. Br Med J 1983;266:1127.)

3. Reduce contractility (beta blockers, Ca^{++}-channel blockers)
4. Dilate coronary arteries (nitrates, Ca^{++}-channel blockers)
5. Reduce afterload (Ca^{++}-channel blockers)

DRUGS FOR THE TREATMENT OF ANGINA PECTORIS

1. Organic Nitrates (Nitroglycerin, Isosorbide Mononitrate, and Isosorbide Dinitrate)

Actions

Organic nitrates stimulate nitrate receptors in the vascular endothelium to increase intracellular cyclic guanosine monophosphate (GMP) formation. The increase in cyclic GMP leads to vascular smooth muscle relaxation by several mechanisms, including

- an inhibition of calcium entry,
- a decreased calcium release from intracellular stores, or
- an increase in calcium extrusion.

As a result of these actions, organic nitrates dilate

- veins (capacitance vessels):
    - to reduce venous return, thereby decreasing left ventricular volume and intramyocardial tension. These actions decrease myocardial oxygen requirements because the major factor controlling the oxygen needs of the heart is the degree to which it is stretched as it fills in diastole.
    - to increase oxygen delivery to the subendocardium. Blood flow to the subendocardium occurs primarily in diastole. By reducing left ventricular end-diastolic pressure, nitrates decrease extravascular compression around the subendocardial vessels and favor a redistribution of coronary blood flow in this area.
- arteries (conductance vessels) to improve regional blood flow to ischemic areas.
- arterioles (precapillary resistance vessels):
    - to decrease peripheral resistance (afterload), thereby reducing the oxygen requirements of the myocardium.
    - to reflexly raise heart rate and increase myocardial oxygen requirements. Fortunately, the increased oxygen demand created by tachycardia is not sufficient to override the beneficial effects of the nitrates which reduce the overall oxygen requirements of the heart.

Uses and Adverse Effects

Various nitrate preparations are available to terminate or prevent anginal attacks. Oral nitroglycerin has an unpredictable effect, due to extensive metabolism during its first pass through the liver in the portal circulation (first-pass metabolism); therefore, other routes must be found for its administration.

- Sublingual nitroglycerin tablets, or nitroglycerin spray applied under or on the tongue, are effective in stopping the pain of angina. If used immediately before an anticipated stress, they can also prevent an attack.
- Topical nitroglycerin patches or ointment are rapidly absorbed through the skin, circumvent first-pass metabolism, and prevent anginal attacks. Because tolerance develops rapidly to the patches if they are applied on a 24-hour basis, they should be applied for only 12 hours per day.
- Buccal nitroglycerin contains nitroglycerin in an inert polymer matrix. This formulation is absorbed through the membranes of the mouth, begins to work promptly, and continues to be effective for a prolonged period.

Isosorbide mononitrate and isosorbide dinitrate, taken orally, are used to prevent anginal attacks.

Headache, due to vasodilatation of the blood vessels in the scalp, is the most common adverse effect of all nitrates.

The other adverse effects are dizziness and weakness, due to postural hypotension when nitrates dilate capacitance vessels.

Tolerance to nitrates develops if vessels are constantly exposed to them. To forestall the development of tolerance, patients should not receive nitrate therapy 24 hours a day.

2. Beta Blockers (Acebutolol, Atenolol, Metoprolol, Nadolol, Propranolol, Timolol)

Actions

The pharmacology of these drugs was presented in Chapter 6.

Beta blockers reduce the oxygen requirements of the heart by decreasing heart rate and force of contraction.

Uses and Adverse Effects

Beta blockers form the mainstay of prophylactic treatment of chronic, stable angina pectoris.

They are often used with a sustained-release nitroglycerin product or isosorbide mononitrate or dinitrate. The combination of a beta blocker with a nitrate is often more effective than either drug used alone. Furthermore, beta blockers prevent the reflex tachycardia that often accompanies nitrate therapy.

The adverse effects and contraindications of beta blockers can be found in Chapter 6.

3. Calcium Channel Blockers/Calcium Entry Blockers (Diltiazem, Felodipine, Isradipine, Nicardipine, Nifedipine, Verapamil)

Actions

Vasoconstriction depends on the entry of small amounts of calcium into the vascular smooth muscle through the calcium channel. Calcium channel blockers (calcium entry blockers) block the entry of calcium into the vascular muscle and prevent vasoconstriction.

All calcium channel blockers dilate coronary vessels, increasing the oxygen supply to patients with variant angina pectoris.

Calcium channel blockers differ, however, in other important respects. These drugs can be divided into the following groups:

- Diltiazem
- The dihydropyridines (amlodipine, felodipine, isradipine, nifedipine, and nicardipine)
- Verapamil

Table 10–1 summaries the cardiovascular effects of these three groups of calcium channel blockers.

Table 10–1
Cardiovascular Effects of Calcium Channel Blockers*

	Dihydropyridines	Diltiazem	Verapamil
Blood pressure	–	–	–
Vasodilatation	+++	++	++
Heart rate	++	–	+/–
Contractility	0/+	0	0/–
Coronary vascular resistance	–	–	–
Blood flow	+++	+++	++

+ = increase; – = decrease; 0 = no significant effect. The magnitude of the response is indicated by the number of symbols.(After Swamy VC, Triggle DJ. Calcium Channel Blockers. In: Craig CR, *Changes are those commonly seen following oral doses in the treatment of hypertension or angina.
Stitzel RE, eds. Modern pharmacology. 4th ed. Boston: Little, Brown, 1994:251.)

The dihydropyridines (amlodipine, felodipine, isradipine, nifedipine, and nicardipine):

- dilate arterioles, decrease peripheral resistance, reduce left ventricular afterload, and decrease myocardial oxygen requirement;
- increase heart rate in response to the fall in peripheral resistance. This effect increases myocardial oxygen requirements, but is sufficiently offset by the other actions of these drugs; and
- frequently do not depress myocardial contractility. All calcium channel blockers directly depress myocardial contractility, but this effect is usually offset in the dihydropyridines by reflex sympathetic stimulation triggered by the fall in peripheral resistance.

Verapamil:

- is a potent myocardial depressant in isolated muscle preparations but produces only mildly decreased contractility in patients with normal cardiac function;
- owes its major anti-anginal effect to peripheral vasodilatation, which decreases afterload and reduces myocardial oxygen demand;
- is also a potent inhibitor of coronary artery spasm and increases myocardial oxygen delivery in patients with variant angina;
- can produce mild bradycardia, increasing the time spent in diastole, when most of the coronary perfusion occurs; and
- does not produce the reflex tachycardia characteristic of the dihydropyridines because verapamil's cardiodepressant effects counterbalance any reflex sympathetic stimulation produced by the decrease in peripheral resistance.

Diltiazem:

- is a less potent peripheral vasodilator than the dihydropyridines;
- is a less potent negative inotrope and chronotrope than verapamil;
- owes its antianginal effects to its ability to
  - ◆ relax the peripheral arterioles, thereby reducing afterload and myocardial oxygen requirements, and
  - ◆ dilate epicardial and subendocardial arteries and inhibit spontaneous coronary spasm, thus increasing oxygen delivery to heart muscle; and
- may also reduce resting heart rate (although generally less than verapamil), which will also increase the time for coronary perfusion.

Uses and Adverse Effects

Calcium channel blockers alleviate the symptoms of variant angina by decreasing the oxygen requirements of the heart and increasing oxygen supply.

In stable angina pectoris, calcium channel blockers reduce myocardial oxygen demand. They decrease the frequency of attacks, reduce nitrate requirements, and improve exercise performance.

A calcium channel blocker may be indicated when nitrates are ineffective or poorly tolerated, or when beta blockers are contraindicated.

Compared to beta blockers, calcium channel blockers

- are preferred in patients with bronchospastic disorders, and
- may be better tolerated in patients with peripheral vascular disease, severe hypertriglyceridemia, or unstable insulin-dependent diabetes mellitus.

The most common adverse effects of the dihydropyridines result from vasodilation. These include headache, flushing and heat sensation, peripheral edema, and hypotension.

Diltiazem's most common adverse effects are nausea, swelling or edema, arrhythmia (atrioventicular [AV] block, bradycardia, tachycardia, and sinus arrest), headache, rash, and fatigue. Diltiazem should be avoided in patients with sick sinus syndrome.

Adverse reactions to verapamil include bradycardia, transient asystole, hypotension, development or worsening of heart failure, development of rhythm disturbances (including AV block and ventricular dysrhythmias), flushing, and peripheral and pulmonary edema. CNS effects include dizziness, headache, fatigue, excitation, vertigo, syncope, and tremor. Constipation, nausea, vomiting and other gastrointestinal complaints are the most common adverse effects seen after oral administration.

11

Antihypertensive Drugs

FACTORS CONTROLLING BLOOD PRESSURE

1. Cardiac output
2. Peripheral resistance

ANTIHYPERTENSIVE DRUGS LOWER BLOOD PRESSURE BY REDUCING CARDIAC OUTPUT OR DECREASING PERIPHERAL RESISTANCE

1. **Reducing cardiac output** with drugs that

   - decrease heart rate and force of contraction (β-blockers), or
   - diminish venous return (venodilators).

2. **Decreasing peripheral resistance** with drugs that

   - reduce renal reabsorption of salt and water (diuretics),
   - dilate arterioles (thiazide and thiazide-like diuretics and vasodilators), or
   - decrease sympathetic centers in the brain (central sympathetic inhibitors).

   Figure 11–1 depicts the sites of action of antihypertensive drugs.

DRUGS THAT REDUCE CARDIAC OUTPUT

1. Beta Blockers (Acebutolol, Atenolol, Metoprolol, Nadolol, Pindolol, Propranolol, Oxprenolol)

Actions (see Chapter 6)

Decrease myocardial contractility and cardiac output.

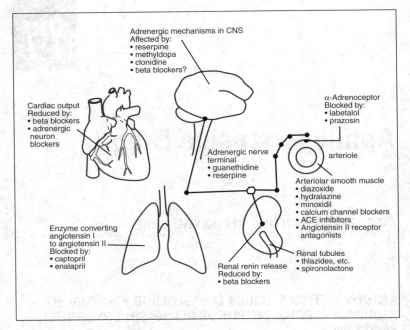

Figure 11–1 Sites of action of antihypertensive drugs. (After O'Brien AJJ, Bulpitt CJ. Anti-hypertensive disease. In: Avery GS, ed. Drug Treatment. 4th ed. Sydney/Auckland: ADIS Press, 1997: 900.)

Reduce renin release, thereby decreasing the formation of angiotensin II and the secretion of aldosterone.

May also reduce sympathetic stimulation within the brain.

Uses and Adverse Effects

Can be used in the first-line treatment of hypertension.

If a beta blocker alone proves inadequate, a diuretic may be added to the treatment regimen.

When the combination of beta blocker and diuretic fails to reduce the hypertension, a vasodilator is usually added as a third drug.

For adverse effects, refer to Chapter 6.

2. Venodilators (Guanethidine and Reserpine)

Actions (see Chapter 6)

Reduce norepinephrine secretion in veins, thereby impairing venous return and decreasing cardiac output.

Decreased sympathetic stimulation of arterioles may also reduce peripheral resistance.

Uses and Adverse Effects

Guanethidine and reserpine are effective antihypertensive drugs, but adverse effects limit their value. When used, these drugs are usually administered with a diuretic, such as hydrochlorothiazide.

For adverse effects, see Chapter 6.

DRUGS THAT DECREASE PERIPHERAL RESISTANCE

1. Diuretics (Thiazides, Chlorthalidone, Metolazone, Furosemide)

Actions (see Chapter 13 and Figure 11–2)

Initially inhibit Na^+, Cl^-, and H_2O reabsorption. As a result, plasma and extracellular fluid (ECF) volumes shrink and cardiac output declines.

With chronic use, plasma volume returns to normal but peripheral resistance decreases.

Vasodilatation is greater with the thiazides, chlorthalidone, and metolazone than with furosemide.

Uses and Adverse Effects

Diuretics are a first-line treatment for hypertension. Because thiazides, chlorthalidone and metolazone dilate arterioles, they are usually preferred

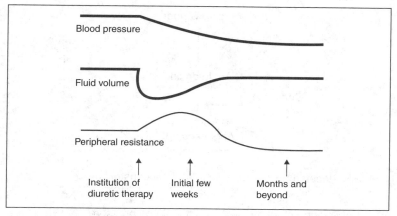

Figure 11–2 Hemodynamic changes responsible for the antihypertensive effects of diuretic therapy. (After Kaplan NM. The therapy of hypertension. In: Kaplan NM, ed. Clinical Hypertension. 4th ed. Baltimore: Williams and Wilkins; 1986:180.)

over furosemide, which does not dilate precapillary resistance vessels, and is not as effective in lowering blood pressure.

If a second drug is necessary, a β-blocker or an ACE inhibitor is frequently added to the diuretic therapy because:

- Diuretics indirectly stimulate β-adrenergic receptors in the kidney to increase the release of renin. The newly released renin is converted first to angiotensin I, which in turn gives rise to angiotensin II, a potent vasoconstrictor. Angiotensin II also releases the mineralocorticoid aldosterone. The action of angiotensin II to constrict arterioles, and the effects of aldosterone to retain salt and water, reduce the antihypertensive effects of diuretics.
- A β-blocker decreases the diuretic-induced increase in renin secretion, thereby increasing the antihypertensive effect of therapy.
- An ACE inhibitor inhibits the conversion of angiotensin I to angiotensin II and reduces the consequences of a diuretic-induced increase in renin. The adverse effects of diuretics are presented in Chapter 13.

2. Vasodilators

A. Angiotensin-Converting Enzyme Inhibitors (Benazepril, Captopril, Cilazapril, Enalapril, Fosinopril, Lisinopril, Quinapril, Ramipril)

Actions (see Chapter 8)

ACE inhibitors reduce the formation of angiotensin II, thereby decreasing peripheral resistance. Refer to Figures 11–3 and 11–4.

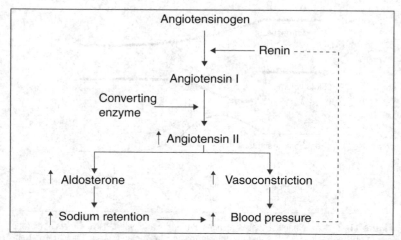

Figure 11–3 Renin-angiotensin-aldosterone axis and blood pressure control. (After Bristol-Myers Squibb.)

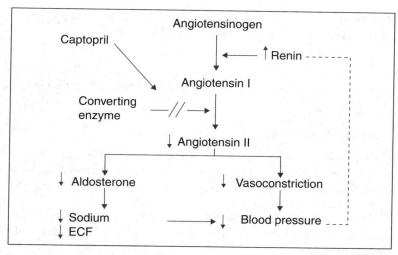

Figure 11–4 Effect of captopril on the renin- angiotensin-aldosterone axis. (After Bristol-Myers Squibb.)

Uses and Adverse Effects

ACE inhibitors are effective alone in treating hypertension.

ACE inhibitors produce fewer adverse effects than other antihypertensives. The alterations in blood chemistry, bradycardia, intermittent claudication, fatigue, cold extremities, and decrease in libido that may be produced by diuretics and β-blockers are not experienced by patients taking ACE inhibitors. However, ACE inhibitors are frequently more expensive than diuretics or β-blockers and this has often relegated them to second-line therapy.

ACE inhibitors may also be combined with a diuretic or a β-blocker.

B. Angiotensin II Receptor Antagonists (Irbesartan, Losartan, Valsartan)

Actions

These drugs block the binding of angiotensin II to type 1 angiotensin II (AT-1) receptors in blood vessels and other tissues.

Uses and Adverse Effects

Angiotensin II receptor antagonists are used alone and in combination with a diuretic for the treatment of hypertension.

Their adverse effects include dizziness and asthenia or fatigue.

C. Calcium Channel Blockers (Amlodipine, Diltiazem, Felodipine, Isradipine, Nicardipine, Nifedipine, and Verapamil)

Actions (see Chapter 10)

These drugs dilate arterioles, decrease peripheral resistance, and lower systemic blood pressure.

Uses and Adverse Effects

Similar to ACE inhibitors, calcium channel blockers (CCBs) are effective antihypertensives and not encumbered by many of the adverse effects commonly associated with the older drugs, such as diuretics, β-blockers, and central sympathetic inhibitors.

However, like ACE inhibitors, CCBs are also frequently more expensive than diuretics or β-blockers and are, therefore, used as second-line treatment of hypertension.

CCB therapy is usually added to initial treatment with a diuretic when the latter agent is not satisfactory alone. Amlodipine, felodipine, isradipine, nicardipine, and nifedipine are often used with a β-blocker. However, verapamil and diltiazem have myocardial depressant effects and are not recommended in combination with beta blocker therapy.

The adverse effects of these drugs were presented in Chapter 10.

D. Hydralazine

Actions

Hydralazine relaxes arteriolar smooth muscles by activating guanylate cyclase, resulting in the accumulation of cyclic guanosine monophosphate (cGMP). The decrease in peripheral resistance increases heart rate and force of contraction, plasma renin activity, and fluid retention.

Hepatic acetylation is the major route for the inactivation of hydralazine. Patients can be divided into rapid acetylators and slow acetylators. During chronic therapy, hydralazine will accumulate in the slow acetylators unless lower doses are given.

Uses and Adverse Effects

The use of hydralazine alone to treat hypertension is limited because of reflex tachycardia.

Hydralazine is often used together with a β-blocker and a diuretic, with the β-blocker preventing tachycardia and the diuretic increasing salt and water excretion.

Hydralazine is contraindicated in patients with coronary artery disease, mitral valvular rheumatic heart disease, and acute dissecting aneurysm of the aorta.

Adverse effects include headache (due to vasodilatation), tachycardia, anginal symptoms, edema, heart failure, anorexia, nausea, dizziness, and sweating. The most serious effect is a lupus erythematosus-like syndrome, most often seen in slow acetylators. These patients must receive lower doses to prevent accumulation of toxic levels of hydralazine.

E. Alpha₁-Adrenergic Blockers (Doxazosin, Prazosin, Terazosin)

Actions (see Chapter 6)

These drugs selectively block α_1-receptors and reduce peripheral resistance.

In contrast to hydralazine, selective α_1-receptor blockers produce only a small increase in heart rate and little change in cardiac output or plasma renin levels.

Uses and Adverse Effects

These drugs are used to treat mild to moderate hypertension.

They are usually taken with a thiazide diuretic and/or other antihypertensive drugs.

For adverse effects, refer to Chapter 6.

F. Alpha₁- and Beta- Receptor Blocker (Labetalol)

Actions (see Chapter 6)

Labetalol blocks both α_1- and β-receptors. Although more potent as a β-blocker, labetalol's antihypertensive effects are due primarily to α_1-blockade, resulting in decreased peripheral resistance.

The reflex bradycardia normally seen with arteriolar dilation is prevented by the partial beta block.

Uses and Adverse Effects

Labetalol is usually added to other therapeutic regimens, notably diuretic therapy.

The adverse effects of labetalol were presented in Chapter 6.

G. Diazoxide and Sodium Nitroprusside

Actions

Diazoxide primarily dilates arterioles. Sodium nitroprusside relaxes both arterioles and veins.

Uses and Adverse Effects

Both drugs are given parenterally to treat hypertensive crises. In this situation, either drug may be lifesaving.

Both drugs are contraindicated in compensatory hypertension, such as that associated with aortic coarctation of AV shunt.

3. Central Sympathetic Inhibitors

A. Clonidine

Actions (see Chapter 6)

Clonidine stimulates α_2-receptors in the brain to inhibit peripheral sympathetic activity. As a result of reduced sympathetic nervous system stimulation, arterioles and veins dilate. In addition, renin release falls.

Uses and Adverse Effects

Clonidine is a very potent antihypertensive. It may be used concomitantly with other antihypertensive agents, such as diuretics or beta blockers.

For adverse effects, refer to Chapter 6.

B. α-Methyldopa (Methyldopa)

Actions (see Chapter 6)

α-Methyldopa reduces central sympathetic activity, decreases total peripheral resistance, and reduces blood pressure. Cardiac output and blood flow are usually maintained in younger patients. In older patients, α-methyldopa may act primarily by dilating veins, thereby reducing preload and cardiac output.

Uses and Adverse Effects

a-Methyldopa is usually employed in a general treatment program in conjunction with a diuretic and/or other antihypertensive drugs. α-Methyldopa may also be used to treat hypertensive crises.

For adverse effects, refer to Chapter 6.

PHARMACOLOGIC APPROACH TO THE TREATMENT OF HYPERTENSION (TABLE 11–1)

Table 11–1

A Protocol for the Treatment of Hypertension with a Diastolic Pressure of 90–120 mm Hg

Step 0	Lifestyle modification, weight loss in the obese, sodium restriction
Step 1	Diuretic (hydrochlorothiazide) or β-blocker
Step 2	Add a β-blocker or diuretic as dictated by drug selected for Step 1 In place of a β-blocker, an ACE inhibitor, angiotensin II receptor antagonist, calcium channel blocker, α_1-blocker, labetalol, or central sympathetic inhibitor may be used
Step 3	Add a vasodilatory such as hydralazine, or α_1-blocker to diuretic plus β-blocker therapy

RATIONALE FOR COMBINATION ANTIHYPERTENSIVE THERAPY (TABLE 11–2)

Guiding Principle

Mild hypertension can often be treated with one antihypertensive. More severe hypertension is often handled by the use of two or more drugs. Drugs should be selected so that they complement each other mechanistically and reduce the consequences of the physiological play-back mechanism evoked by the other agent.

Table 11–2

Rationale for Combining Antihypertensive Drugs

Drug	Physiological Play-Back Mechanism	Appropriate Drugs to Use in Combination
Diuretic	Increase in renin-angiotensin-aldosterone axis	**β-Blocker** — reduces renin release and decreases cardiac output **ACE Inhibitor** — reduces formation of angiotensin II and secretion of aldosterone **Angiotensin II Receptor Antagonist** — blocks the action of released angiotensin II
β-Blocker	Decrease in renal perfusion can increase blood volume	**Diuretic** — decreases blood volume

Continued

Table 11–2
Rationale for Combining Antihypertensive Drugs—Continued

Drug	Physiological Play-Back Mechanism	Appropriate Drugs to Use in Combination
ACE Inhibitor, Angiotensin II Receptor Antagonist, Calcium Channel Blocker (CCB)	No direct play-back mechanisms. ACE inhibitors, angiotensin II receptor antagonists, and CCBs are often combined with other drugs to affect a greater fall in BP	**Diuretic** — often combined with ACE inhibitor or angiotensin II receptor antagonist (see above). Adding a CCB to a diuretic also increases the overall antihypertensive effect **β-Blocker** — often combined with ACE inhibitor, angiotensin III receptor antagonist, or CCB to increase antihypertensive effect
Hydralazine,	Reflex tachycardia and increased myocardial contractility with increased cardiac output. Increased renin release results in angiotensin II-mediated vasoconstriction and aldosterone-mediated fluid retention	**Diuretic** — reduces fluid retention. **β-Blocker** — reduces reflex stimulation of the heart and decreases the release of renin by the kidneys
Central Sympathetic Inhibitor	Decrease in peripheral resistance may result in an increased retention of sodium, chloride, and water	**Diuretic** — increases sodium, chloride, and water excretion. In addition, thiazides, chlorthalidone, and metolazone decrease peripheral resistance
Adrenergic Neuron Blocker	Fall in cardiac output (secondary to reduced venous return), reduces renal perfusion, resulting in sodium, chloride, and water retention	**Diuretic** — increases excretion of salt and water. In addition, thiazides, chlorthalidone, and metolazone decrease peripheral resistance and this effect further reduces blood pressure

12

Drugs for the Treatment of Hypotension and Shock

SHOCK

Shock is a condition of acute peripheral circulatory failure. It can result from the loss of circulating fluid. Therapy is aimed at correcting the hypoperfusion of vital organs. **Hypovolemic shock** is treated by volume replacement; **bacteremic shock** by intensive antibiotic therapy, corticosteroids, and volume replacement. In addition, sympathomimetic drugs or vasodilators (which either increase cardiac output, or alter peripheral resistance, or both) may be appropriate.

TISSUE PERFUSION OF HEART, BRAIN, AND KIDNEYS DURING HYPOTENSION AND SHOCK

Heart and Brain

The major factor regulating blood flow through the coronary and cerebral vessels is the mean diastolic pressure. In the presence of hypotension, myocardial and cerebral perfusion are compromised. In this situation, a sympathomimetic drug that increases blood pressure will improve the perfusion of both the heart and brain. Sympathomimetics can be used without concern of constricting the blood vessels in these organs. The caliber of these vessels is determined by the metabolic needs of the tissue, not by stimulation of adrenergic receptors.

The heart and brain differ from each other with respect to their need for oxygen.

- Although the heart normally uses an aerobic metabolic pathway, it can operate for a short time anaerobically.
- The brain needs oxygen for its metabolism and is particularly susceptible to the consequences of acute hypotension and shock.

107

Kidney

In contrast to the heart and brain, the kidney extracts only a relatively small amount of the oxygen provided to it under resting conditions. This means it can withstand, within limits, a reduction in blood flow by extracting a higher percentage of the oxygen supplied.

However, sympathetic stimulation causes renal vasoconstriction. Adrenergic vasoconstrictors also reduce blood flow, possibly leading to renal ischemia.

SYMPATHOMIMETICS

Sympathomimetics are used to improve tissue perfusion. They stimulate

1. α_1-receptors, to increase venous return and peripheral resistance;
2. β_1-receptors, to increase heart rate and cardiac output (if venous return is adequate); or
3. dopamine receptors, to dilate the renal and splanchnic beds.

1. Epinephrine (Adrenaline)

Actions (see Chapter 5)

Epinephrine stimulates β_1-receptors in the heart to increase both heart rate and force of contraction. In small doses, epinephrine stimulates

- β_2-receptors on arterioles (precapillary resistance vessels) in skeletal muscles to decrease peripheral resistance, and
- α_1-receptors on veins to increase venous return.

Larger doses of epinephrine stimulate α_1-receptors on arterioles throughout the body to produce a generalized vasoconstriction and an increase in peripheral resistance.

Epinephrine also dilates bronchioles.

Uses and Adverse Effects

Epinephrine is the drug of choice to treat anaphylactic shock because it antagonizes the effects of histamine, which constricts bronchioles and dilates blood vessels.

- By stimulating β_2-receptors, epinephrine prevents or reverses histamine-induced bronchoconstriction.
- By stimulating α_1-receptors, epinephrine reverses histamine-induced vasodilatation.

For the adverse effects of epinephrine, refer to Chapter 5.

2. Levarterenol (Norepinephrine and Noradrenaline)

Actions (see Chapter 5)

Levarterenol stimulates α_1-receptors, constricting both capacitance and precapillary resistance vessels (veins and arterioles). The resulting increase in blood pressure activates the carotid sinus and aortic arch pressor receptors to reflexly stimulate the vagus nerve. The result is a fall in heart rate and cardiac output.

Uses and Adverse Effects

Levarterenol is indicated for the maintenance of blood pressure in acute hypotensive states, surgical and nonsurgical trauma, central vasomotor depression, and hemorrhage.

For adverse effects, refer to Chapter 5.

3. Dobutamine and Dopamine

Refer to Chapter 5 for information on these drugs.

VASODILATORS

Vasodilators are used in patients with severe pump failure following acute myocardial infarction and in individuals with refractory chronic congestive heart failure. Vasodilators

1. increase cardiac output by reducing peripheral resistance (afterload reduction),
2. relieve pulmonary congestion by increasing venous capacitance (preload reduction), and
3. limit the extent of ischemic damage by reducing myocardial oxygen demand and increasing myocardial oxygen supply.

1. Sodium Nitroprusside

Actions (see Chapter 8)

Nitroprusside dilates venous and arterial beds. Because it has a greater effect on afterload than nitroglycerin, nitroprusside is more likely to increase cardiac output.

Uses and Adverse Effects

Nitroprusside can be used to treat severe persistent pump failure in patients with markedly reduced cardiac output and increased peripheral resistance.

Nitroprusside is particularly valuable in patients with severe acute decompensated chronic congestive heart failure, refractory to digoxin and diuretics.

Nitroprusside should not be used in the treatment of compensatory hypertension, eg, AV shunt or coarctation of the aorta.

For adverse effects, refer to Chapter 8.

2. Intravenous Nitroglycerin

Actions

Nitroglycerin dilates both arterial and venous vessels, with a greater effect on the venous side.

Intravenous (IV) nitroglycerin relieves pulmonary congestion, decreases myocardial oxygen consumption, and reduces ST segment elevation.

Uses and Adverse Effects

IV nitroglycerin can be used to decrease myocardial ischemia and improve hemodynamics in severe left ventricular dysfunction complicating acute myocardial infarction.

Its primary use is in patients with recurrent ischemic pain, or in patients with marked elevation of left ventricular filling pressure and pulmonary edema.

Major adverse effects include symptomatic hypotension, reflex tachycardia, paradoxical increase of anginal pain, and palpitation.

Central nervous system effects include transient headache, weakness, dizziness, apprehension, and restlessness.

Patients may also experience nausea, vomiting, abdominal pain, and methemoglobinemia.

13

Diuretics

REABSORPTION OF SODIUM, CHLORIDE, AND WATER FROM THE NEPHRON (FIGURE 13–1 AND TABLES 13–1 AND 13–2)

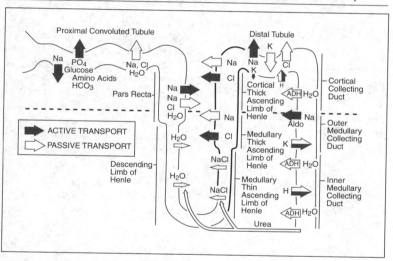

Figure 13–1 The reabsorption of electrolytes and water from the nephron. ADH = antidiuretic hormone. (After Jacobson HR, Kokko JR. Diuretics, sites and mechanisms of action. Ann Rev Pharmacol Toxicol 1976; 16:201–204.)

Table 13–1

Percent of Filtered Water and Sodium Remaining in Different Segments of the Nephron

Segment of Nephron	% H$_2$O Remaining	% Na$^+$ Remaining
End of proximal tubule	20	20
End of loop of henle	14	7
End of distal tubule	2 – 5	1 – 5
Excreted urine	0.1 – 1	0 – 1

Table 13–2

Reabsorption of Sodium, Chloride, Bicarbonate, and Water and Secretion of Potassium and Hydrogen Ions in Different Segments of the Nephron

	Proximal Tubule	Ascending Limb of Loop of Henle	Distal Tubule	Collecting Ducts
Na^+	Active	Passive; follows Cl^-	Active, exchanged for K^+ and H^+. Aldosterone is responsible for the exchange of K^+ and H^+ for Na^+; CA controls an exchange of H^+ for Na^+	Active, exchanged for K^+ and H^+. Aldosterone is responsible for the exchange of K^+ and H^+ for Na^+; CA controls an exchange of H^+ for Na^+
Cl^-	Passive, follows Na^+	Active, taking Na^+ with it	1. Some Cl^- ions are reabsorbed passively with Na^+. 2. Other Cl^- ions are retained in the tubular lumen to electrically balance K^+ that is secreted in exchange for re-absorbed Na^+ ions	1. Some Cl^- ions are reabsorbed passively with Na^+. 2. Other Cl^- ions are retained in the tubular lumen to electrically balance K^+ that is secreted in exchange for reabsorbed Na^+ ions
K^+			Secreted into tubule in exchange for Na^+	Secreted into tubule in exchange for Na^+
H^+	Secreted into tubule in exchange for Na^+, then reabsorbed CA involved		Secreted into tubule in exchange for Na^+	Secreted into tubule in exchange for Na^+
HCO_3^-	Reabsorbed; depends on CA		Reabsorbed; depends on CA	Reabsorbed, depends on CA
H_2O	Passive; follows NA^+	Ascending limb is impermeable to H_2O, which stays in tubular lumen	Passive; follows Na^+	Passive; into hypertonic medulla in presence of ADH

CA = carbonic anhydrase; ADH = antidiuretic hormone.

FACTORS INFLUENCING THE REABSORPTION OF SODIUM AND WATER IN THE NEPHRON

Carbonic Anhydrase

Carbonic anhydrase (CA) catalyzes the reaction:

$$H_2O + CO_2 \rightleftharpoons H^+ + HCO_3^-$$

Carbonic anhydrase

- provides H^+ for exchange with Na^+, and
- promotes:
    - reabsorption of Na^+, HCO_3^-, and H^+ in the proximal tubule,
    - secretion of H^+ in the distal tubule and collecting duct, and
    - reabsorption of fixed base. HCO_3^- formed in the proximal tubule is reabsorbed, retaining fixed base.

Inhibiting CA increases

- HCO_3^- excretion,
- urine pH, and
- K^+ excretion (in the absence of H^+, more K^+ is exchanged for Na^+).

Aldosterone

Under the influence of aldosterone, Na^+ in the distal tubule and collecting duct is reabsorbed in exchange for K^+ and H^+, which are secreted into the tubular lumen. Aldosterone antagonists block this exchange, increase Na^+ excretion, and decrease the loss of K^+ and H^+ ions.

Antidiuretic Hormone

In the presence of antidiuretic hormone (ADH), collecting ducts are permeable to H_2O, which is reabsorbed into the hypertonic medulla. In the absence of ADH, water cannot be reabsorbed from collecting ducts and the kidney excretes a dilute urine.

Impermeability of the Ascending Limb of the Loop of Henle to H_2O

The inability of water to follow Na^+ and Cl^- from the ascending limb of the loop of Henle into the medulla of the kidney is essential to the formation of a hypertonic medulla. It is the presence of a hypertonic medulla that facilitates the final concentration of urine when water in the collecting ducts is drawn into the medulla. The hypertonic medulla also depends on the reabsorption of urea from the collecting ducts.

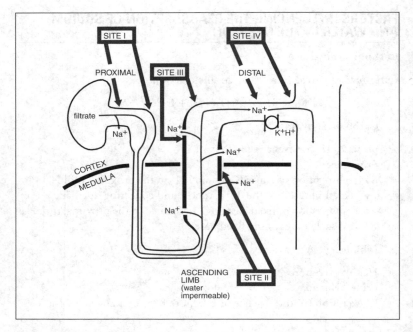

Figure 13–2 Sites of sodium reabsorption and diuretic action in the nephron. I = proximal tubule; II = ascending limb of Henle's loop; III = cortical diluting site; IV = distal Na⁺/K⁺H⁺ exchange site. (After Lant AF, Wilson GM. Modern diuretic therapy. Physiological basis and practical aspects. Excerpta Medica 1974:7.)

SITES OF ACTION OF DIURETICS WITHIN THE NEPHRON (FIGURE 13–2 AND TABLE 13–3)
GROUPS OF DIURETICS

1. Thiazides, Chlorthalidone, and Metolazone

Actions

These drugs block Na^+ and Cl^- reabsorption in the cortical diluting segment of the loop of Henle (site III) and in the proximal section of the distal convoluted tubule (site IV). Water is retained in the nephron because of the osmotic drawing power of Na^+ and Cl^-. These drugs do not alter the hypertonicity of the renal medulla or reduce the capacity of the nephron to concentrate urine in the collecting ducts. Because of increased Na^+ arriving in the distal tubules and collecting ducts, more K^+ is secreted in exchange. This can lead to hypokalemia.

Uses

These drugs are used as adjunct therapy in congestive heart failure, hepatic cirrhosis, corticosteroid and estrogen therapy, and edema of renal origin.

Table 13–3

Consequences of Reducing Sodium Reabsorption in Different Segments of the Nephron

Site	Consequence
I = Proximal tubule	Although most of the glomerular filtrate is reabsorbed in the proximal tubule, drugs which impair salt and water reabsorption here have little effect on urine production because salt and water retained in the proximal tubule are reabsorbed in the subsequent portions of the nephron
II = Ascending limb of Henle's loop	Loop diuretics inhibit sodium and chloride reabsorption from site II, reduce the hypertonicity of the medulla, and prevent the final concentration of urine in the collecting ducts
III = Cortical diluting site	Drugs that block the reabsorption of sodium and chloride at site III (cortical diluting segment) produce a marked diuresis. They are not as potent as loop diuretics because they do not modify the hypertonicity of the renal medulla or the concentrating ability of the collecting ducts
IV = Distal Na^+/K^+ H^+ exchange site	Most of the salt and water filtered through the glomeruli is reabsorbed before it reaches the distal convoluted tubule. Drugs that work at site IV have only limited effectiveness. Potassium-sparing diuretics work in the distal tubules and collecting ducts to reduce the secretion of K^+ in exchange for Na^+

Also used in the treatment of hypertension (see Chapter 11).

Adverse Effects

Hypovolemia, hyponatremia, hypokalemia, hyperuricemia with attacks of gout, hyperglycemia due to decreased insulin release.

2. Loop Diuretics (Furosemide, Ethacrynic Acid, Bumetanide)

Actions

Loop diuretics inhibit Cl^- reabsorption in the ascending limb of the loop of Henle in the renal medulla (site II). Na^+ remains with Cl^- in the tubular lumen to maintain electrical neutrality. The resulting reduction in hypertonicity in the medulla impairs the urine-concentrating ability of the collecting ducts.

Uses

Loop diuretics are used in the treatment of edema in patients with severe edema or renal impairment in which thiazides, chlorthalidone, or metolazone are ineffective.

Also used in the treatment of hypertension; however, thiazides, chlorthalidone, or metolazone are usually preferred because loop diuretics do not dilate arterioles (see Chapter 11).

Adverse Effects

Electrolyte depletion, manifested as weakness, dizziness, lethargy, leg cramps, sweating, bladder spasms, anorexia, or mental confusion.

Hyperuricemia and attacks of gout, Dermatitis, rashes, Vertigo, tinnitus, reversible deafness.

3. Potassium-Sparing Diuretics

A. Spironolactone

Actions

Spironolactone competitively blocks aldosterone receptors in the distal convoluted tubule (site IV).

Uses

Spironolactone is used in the treatment of conditions of excessive aldosterone levels, primary aldosteronism, and cirrhosis. Treatment of congestive heart failure.

Combined with a thiazide diuretic, chlorthalidone, metolazone, or a loop diuretic to prevent diuretic-induced hypokalemia.

Adverse Effects

Hyperkalemia, gynecomastia, nausea, cramping diarrhea.

B. Triamterene and Amiloride

Actions

Triamterene and amiloride act directly on tubular transport in the distal convoluted tubules and collecting ducts to inhibit Na^+ reabsorption and K^+ secretion. Actions are independent of aldosterone.

Uses

Triamterene and amiloride are used in the treatment of edema associated with congestive heart failure, cirrhosis, nephrotic syndrome, steroid-induced edema, and edema secondary to hyperaldosteronism.

Primary use of these drugs is with a thiazide diuretic, chlorthalidone, metolazone, or loop diuretic to reduce or prevent diuretic-induced hypokalemia.

Adverse Effects

Hyperkalemia.

4. Osmotic Diuretics (Mannitol)

Actions

Osmotic diuretics are pharmacologically inert electrolytes. They are freely filtered by the glomerulus and not reabsorbed. When excreted, they carry an amount of water equivalent to their osmotic drawing power.

Uses

Mannitol is used to increase urine production when the glomerular filtration rate (GFR) is acutely reduced. In this situation, loop diuretics cannot reduce the reabsorbing capacity of the nephron sufficiently to increase urine flow.

Also used to reduce cerebrospinal fluid volume and pressure.

Adverse Effects

Increased extracellular fluid volume. Hypersensitivity reactions.

Part 4 Drugs and the Blood

14

Antihyperlipidemic Drugs

RATIONALE FOR LOWERING PLASMA LIPIDS

Myocardial Infarction

Caused by atherosclerosis. Is the most common cause of death in the Western world.

Three Factors Implicated in Atherosclerosis

1. Hypertension
2. Smoking
3. High plasma lipids

Rationale for Antihyperlipidemic Drugs

1. Antihyperlipidemic drugs reduce elevated plasma lipids
2. Decreasing plasma lipid levels reduces the risk of myocardial infarcts

CLASSIFICATION OF PLASMA LIPOPROTEINS (TABLE 14–1)

Table 14–1
Comparative Classification of Plamsa Lipoproteins

Ultracentrifugation		Electrophoresis
1. Chylomicrons, found near the top of tube. Contain 80–90% triglycerides (TG)	=	Band that remains at the origin of the electrophoresis plate
2. Very-low-density lipoproteins (VLDL). Contain 50–70% TG and 20% cholesterol	=	Prebeta band, moves slowly down the electrophoresis plate

Continued

Table 14–1

Comparative Classification of Plamsa Lipoproteins—Continued

Ultracentrifugation	Electrophoresis
3. Low-density lipoproteins (LDL) Responsible for 75% of cholesterol found in plasma	= Beta band, moves farther down the electrophoresis plate than the prebeta band
4. High-density lipoproteins (HDL), found near bottom of tube. Contain about 20% cholesterol and 8% TG. An inverse relationship exists between HDL levels and incidence of coronary heart disease in subjects over age 50	= Alpha lipoproteins, move farthest down the electrophoresis plate

ORIGINS OF PLASMA LIPOPROTEINS (FIGURE 14–1)

Chylomicrons

Formed in the intestines from food. They mainly contain triglycerides synthesized from fatty acids, with more than 12 carbons, and cholesterol. Once absorbed into the lymph and transported to the plasma, chylomicrons are acted on by lipoprotein lipase, an enzyme located at the endothelial surface of capillary blood vessels. This enzyme releases triglycerides, which are subsequently stored as fat or converted to fatty acids. The remaining chylomicron remnant particles, rich in cholesterol of dietary origin, are bound and internalized in liver cells, and then degraded by lysosomal enzymes. This process delivers cholesterol of dietary origin to the liver.

VLDL

VLDL, containing 50 to 70% triglycerides and 20% cholesterol, are formed in the liver from free fatty acids (FFA), cholesterol, and carbohydrate. VLDL are stripped of some of their triglycerides by lipoprotein lipase and converted to intermediate-density lipoproteins (IDL).

LDL

Formed from IDL as the latter lose triglycerides. LDL contain mainly cholesterol. They are removed from the circulation through binding with plasma membrane B-100/E receptor (the LDL receptor) in the liver and extrahepatic tissues. Most LDL appear to be removed by the liver. A deficiency of LDL-receptor activity results in type IIa hypercholesterolemia, also known as familial hypercholesterolemia.

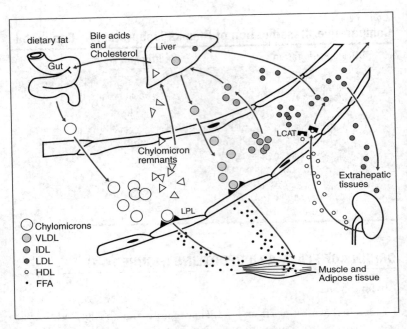

Figure 14–1 Schematic overview of lipoprotein transport and turnover. VLDL = very-low-density lipoproteins; IDL = intermediate-density lipoproteins; LDL = low-density lipoproteins; HDL = high-density lipoproteins; FFA = free fatty acids; LPL = lipoprotein lipase; LCAT = lecithin:cholesterol acyltransferase. (After Forster C. Hyerlipoproteinemia and antihyperlipidemic drugs. In: Kalant H, Roschlau W, eds. Principles of Medical Pharmacology. 5th ed. Toronto: B.C. Decker, 1989:375–385.)

HDL

The precursors of HDL (nascent HDL) are produced by the liver and converted to mature HDL in the circulation as a result of acquiring cholesterol ester and apoproteins from other lipoproteins. HDL play a role in the metabolism of chylomicrons and VLDL. HDL could also be important for the transport of cholesterol out of peripheral tissues (including arterioles) to the liver for disposal. This reverse cholesterol transport could be the basis for the inverse correlation between coronary heart disease and plasma HDL levels.

CAUSES OF HYPERLIPIDEMIAS

Hyperlipidemias may be of exogenous or endogenous origin (Table 14–2).

Table 14–2
Causes of Hyperlipidemias

Exogenous Hyperlipidemia	Exogenous hyperlipidemia results from the ingestion of a meal high in fatty acids containing 12 or more carbons. The chylomicrons formed are released into the circulation by the intestinal lymphatics. Exogenous hyperlipidemia can be reduced by eating food containing fatty acids having fewer than 12 carbons, because they are absorbed directly into the portal circulation and carried to the liver
Endogenous Hyperlipidemia	Endogenous hyperlipidemia results from an increase in the synthesis of lipoproteins or a decrease in their rate of removal from the plasma. Excessive hepatic triglyceride and VLDL synthesis in the liver is the most common cause of hypertriglyceridemia. Triglyceride synthesis is stimulated by caloric excess, dietary carbohydrates, ethanol, estrogens, and hyperinsulinism secondary to peripheral insulin antagonism, such as is seen in obesity and corticosteroid excess. Endogenous hypertriglyceridemia may also be genetic in origin
	Lipoprotein lipase is responsible for the removal of triglycerides from VLDL and chylomicrons. A defect in this enzyme is the most common cause of massive hypertriglyceridemia. Both insulin and thyroxin are required for the maintenance of lipoprotein lipase activity. Uncontrolled diabetes mellitus and hypothyroidism are the leading causes of severe hypertriglyceridemia. Treatment with insulin or thyroid hormone reverses the condition
	Endogenous hypercholesterolemia can result from overproduction of cholesterol in the liver. This condition is associated with obesity and genetic abnormalities and can result in premature coronary heart disease

TREATMENT OF HYPERLIPIDEMIAS

Initial Non-Drug Treatment

Initial treatment for hyperlipidemia should include a specific diet, weight reduction, and an exercise program. Patients with diabetes mellitus must maintain good diabetic control. Drug therapy is often not recommended until diet and exercise have been tried for two to three months. The institution of drug therapy should not mean that non-drug therapy be discontinued. Nonpharmacologic means of hyperlipidemia control must remain an integral part of the treatment regimen.

DRUG TREATMENT

1. Drugs Primarily Affecting VLDL

The Fibrates (Benzafibrate, Clofibrate, Fenofibrate, Gemfibrozil)

Actions

The mechanism of action of the fibrates has not been established, but likely involves

- catabolism of VLDL, as a result of increased lipoprotein and hepatic triglyceride lipase activity; and
- attenuation of triglyceride biosynthesis by acetyl-coenzyme A (CoA) carboxylase inhibition.

Fibrates decrease both LDL and VLDL. However, because their major action is to increase lipoprotein and hepatic triglyceride lipase, fibrates produce a greater reduction of VLDL.

Uses

Fibrates are used to treat patients with hypercholesterolemia of types

- IIa (hyperbetalipoproteinemia), characterized by increased LDL, normal VLDL, and absence of chylomicrons; and
- IIb (combined or mixed hyperlipidemia), characterized by increased LDL, increased VLDL, and absence of chylomicrons.

Adverse Effects

Fibrates are generally well tolerated. Most common immediate adverse effects are abdominal discomfort, epigastric fullness, nausea, and mild diarrhea.

Fibrates may potentiate the effects of sulfonylurea hypoglycemics and warfarin.

2. Drugs Primarily Affecting LDL

A. The Resins (Cholestyramine and Colestipol)

Actions

Cholestyramine and colestipol are nonabsorbed resins that sequester bile acids in the intestine, preventing their absorption. The liver responds to the lowered levels of bile acids by increasing the conversion of cholesterol to bile acids, thereby lowering cholesterol levels and increasing LDL-receptor activity and apoprotein B catabolism.

Unfortunately, the decrease in LDL is partly offset by a compensatory increase in cholesterol synthesis in the liver and intestine.

Uses

Cholestyramine and colestipol are used to treat hyperlipidemias characterized by an increase in beta lipoproteins or LDL.

They are used in situations where the increase is seen in LDL alone or where the increase in LDL is accompanied by a rise in VLDL.

Adverse Effects

Cholestyramine and colestipol's adverse effects include abdominal discomfort, bloating, nausea, dyspepsia, steatorrhea, and possibly either constipation or diarrhea.

Cholestyramine and colestipol bind to acidic drugs (including warfarin, phenylbutazone, digoxin, thiazides, phenobarbital, and thyroid hormones) in the GI tract, thereby decreasing their absorption.

Cholestyramine and colestipol also block the absorption of fat-soluble vitamins and tetracycline antibiotics.

B. The Statins (Atorvastatin Fluvastatin, Lovastatin, Pravastatin, Simvastatin)

Actions

The statins reduce LDL synthesis by inhibiting 3-hydroxy-3-methylglutaryl-coenzyme A (HMG-CoA) reductase. This enzyme catalyzes the conversion of HMG-CoA to mevalonate, which is an early and rate-limiting step in the biosynthesis of cholesterol.

The statins also increase LDL catabolism, as a result of the induction of LDL receptors.

They may also increase HDL levels.

Uses

The statins are used to reduce elevated cholesterol levels in patients with primary hypercholesterolemia of type IIa and IIb.

Adverse Effects

Most common complaints at the start of therapy are nausea, epigastric fullness, distension, constipation or loose bowel actions, and headache.

Mild elevations in liver enzymes (transaminases) are common and exceed the apparent safe level (3x the normal upper limit) in about 1.5% of patients. Liver function should therefore be monitored every 4 to 6 weeks during the first year of therapy and periodically thereafter.

A combination of muscle weakness and raised plasma creatine phosphokinase levels affects approximately 1 to 2 patients for every 1000 taking statins. On rare occasions, this has been reported to progress to rhabdomyolysis and myoglobinuria. It is believed that the risk of myopathy is greater when HMG-CoA reductase inhibitors are administered concurrently with cyclosporine, erythromycin, gemfibrozil, or nicotinic acid.

Cholestyramine and colestipol may decrease the bioavailability of statins. If combined therapy is required, give the statin at least 1 hour before or 4 hours after cholestyramine or colestipol.

3. Miscellaneous Drugs

A. Niacin (Nicotinic Acid)

Actions

Niacin reduces triglyceride synthesis, thereby decreasing hepatic secretion of VLDL.

This action of niacin may be explained by its ability to inhibit lipolysis in adipose tissue, which lowers FFA and decreases the hepatic synthesis of triglycerides. This is because circulating FFA, derived almost totally from adipose tissue, are the main source of fatty acids for the synthesis of triglycerides in the liver.

Since LDL is derived from VLDL, a reduction of plasma VLDL concentration can lead to a decrease in circulating levels of LDL, and thus of cholesterol.

Uses

Niacin is used effectively for the treatment of both hypercholesterolemias and hypertriglyceridemias. Therefore, it has value in the treatment of type IIb hyperlipoproteinemia, in which both VLDL and LDL are increased.

Niacin may also increase HDL.

Adverse Effects

The most common and annoying adverse reaction is the development of an intense cutaneous flush and pruritus that severely limits compliance with the drug. However, with continued use, these symptoms will disappear in most patients.

Gastrointestinal distress is often encountered with niacin therapy but can be decreased by taking the drug with meals and using antacids.

More severe, but less frequent, side effects of niacin include abnormal liver function tests, decreased glucose tolerance, glycosuria, hyperuricemia, and jaundice.

Niacin is contraindicated in patients with hepatic dysfunction, active peptic ulcers, or hyperuricemia. It should be used with caution in patients with diabetes mellitus, since it can result in deterioration of blood glucose control in non–insulin-dependent patients.

B. Probucol

Actions

The mechanism of action of probucol is not known, but may be related to increased catabolism of LDL.

Probucol reduces total cholesterol and LDL-cholesterol concentrations without substantially affecting serum VLDL-cholesterol or triglyceride levels.

Uses

Probucol is used in the treatment of patients with elevated LDL or combined hyperlipidemias.

Adverse Effects

Probucol's adverse effects are diarrhea, flatulence, abdominal pain, and nausea.

15

Anticoagulant and Antiplatelet Drugs, Fibrinolytic Agents, and Vitamin K

THROMBI AND EMBOLI

Groups of Drugs Used in the Management of Thrombi and Emboli

1. Anticoagulants, which inhibit the formation of fibrin
2. Antiplatelet drugs, which reduce platelet adhesion and aggregation
3. Fibrinolytic and thrombolytic agents, which digest fibrin

Formation of Venous and Arterial Thrombi

Venous thrombi usually form in regions of slow or disturbed blood flow. They begin as small deposits in either the valve cusp pockets or the venous sinuses of the deep veins of the legs.

Coagulation of the blood plays a major role in the formation and extension of venous thrombi.

Arterial thrombi are formed after damage to the endothelium of the artery, which allows platelets to adhere to the vessel wall and serve as the focus for thrombus formation (Figure 15–1). The adhesion of a few platelets to the vessel wall is followed by the aggregation of increased numbers of thrombocytes. Fibrin, formed by coagulation, subsequently encases the platelets, giving rise to a platelet-fibrin plug. Because blood flow in the arteries is rapid, arterial thrombi stay close to vessel walls and have been termed **mural thrombi**. A mural thrombus may either remain at its original site or

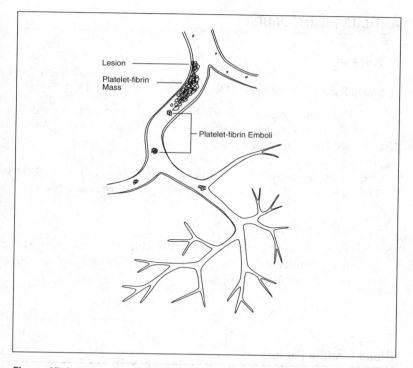

Figure 15–1 Diagrammatic representation of platelet adhesion in formation of arterial emboli. (After Mustard JF, Packham MA. Platelets, thrombosis and drugs. Drugs 1975; 9:25.)

be sheared away by the rapid blood flow to locate in other parts of the body. If it remains at its site of origin, the mural thrombus can serve as a focus for further platelet aggregation. In that case, a platelet-fibrin plug may be formed, which becomes incorporated into the vessel wall to produce atherosclerosis-like lesions.

Anticoagulants

Used to prevent thrombus formation in the veins, where coagulation plays an important role.

Antiplatelet Drugs

Used to stop microemboli from forming in the arteries and arterioles, where platelet adhesion plays an important role.

ANTICOAGULANT DRUGS

1. Heparin

Actions (Table 15–1 and Figure 15–2)

Works by means of a plasma cofactor, the heparin cofactor, or antithrombin III which neutralizes several activated clotting factors: XIIa, kallikrein, XIa, IXa, Xa, IIA, and XIIIa.

Has an immediate but fleeting anticoagulant effect.

Decreases plasma turbidity by stimulating the release of a lipase from capillary walls which breaks down chylomicrons and free fatty acids.

Uses

Prevents new clot formation and limits propagation of existing thrombi.

Effects are monitored by coagulation tests, such as whole blood clotting time, thrombin time, or activated partial thromboplastin time (aPTT).

Table 15–1
Blood Clotting Factors

Factor	Common Synonyms	Factor	Common Synonyms
I	Fibrinogen	IX	Christmas factor, plasma thromboplastin component (PTC)
I'	Fibrin monomer	X	Stuart factor
I"	Fibrin polymer	XI	Plasma thromboplastin antecedent (PTA)
II	Prothrombin	XII	Hageman factor
III	Tissue thromboplastin	XIII	Fibrin-stabilizing factor (FSF)
IV	Calcium, Ca^{++}	HMW-K	High-molecular-weight kininogen, Fitzgerald factor
V	Labile factor	Pre-K	Prekallikrein, Fletcher factor
VII	Proconvertin	Ka	Kallikrein
VIII	Antihemophilic globulin (AHG)	PL	Platelet phospholipid

(After O'Reilly RA. Anticoagulant, antithrombotic, and thrombolytic drugs. In: Gilman AG, Goodman LS, Rall TW, Murad F, eds. The pharmacological basis of therapeutics. 7th ed. New York: MacMillan, 1985:1338.)

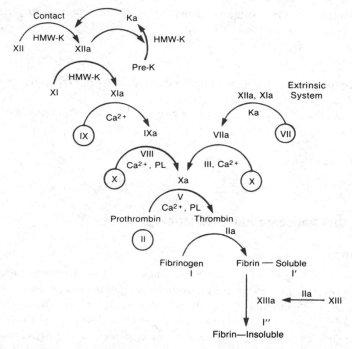

Figure 15–2 Intrinsic and extrinsic systems of blood coagulation. (After O'Reilly RA. Anticoagulant, antithrombotic, and thrombolytic drugs. In: Gilman AG, Goodman LS, Rall TW, Murad F, eds. The pharmacological basis of therapeutics. 7th ed. New York: MacMillan, 1985:1338.)

Adverse Effects

Hemorrhage, local irritation, mild pain or hematoma at site of injection, hypersensitivity, osteoporosis, alopecia, thrombocytopenia, aldosterone suppression.

2. Low-Molecular-Weight Heparins (Dalteparin, and Enoxaparin)

Actions

Derived from heparin by depolymerization, low-molecular-weight heparins differ from unfractionated heparin in their high ratio of antifactor Xa to antifactor IIa (antithrombin) activity, producing a more favourable ratio of antithrombotic effect to bleeding risk.

Have greater bioavailability than unfractionated heparin, permitting fewer daily doses, more predictable plasma heparin concentrations, and subcutaneous administration of fixed dosages without monitoring plasma antifactor Xa activity or aPTT.

Uses

Used in prophylaxis of thromboembolic disorders (deep vein thrombosis) and in surgery.

Compared to heparin, they have a reduced likelihood of causing hemorrhage.

Adverse Effects

Hemorrhage.

3. Oral Anticoagulants (Warfarin)

Actions

Prevents formation of new fibrin thrombi and reduces extension of already formed clots, by competitively antagonizing vitamin K thereby preventing hepatic synthesis of the biologically active forms of the vitamin K–dependent clotting factors II, VII, IX, and X (indicated by circles in Figure 15–2).

Delayed onset of action. Effect not evident until the active factors already present in blood are catabolized, ranging from 5 hours for factor VII to 2 to 3 days for factor II.

Initially prolongs one-stage prothrombin time by depressing factor VII levels.

Effects depend on reduction of all four vitamin K–dependent clotting factors.

Uses

To treat acute deep vein thrombosis, rheumatic valve disease, and patients recovering from myocardial infarcts or suffering from cerebrovascular disease.

Effects controlled by prothrombin time (PT) are reported in terms of an international normalized ratio (INR). The observed PT is corrected depending on the reagent used in the testing. For most situations, the target INR is 2 to 3.

Adverse Effects

Hemorrhage. Drug interactions are common with warfarin. Consult an appropriate reference source for a list of the drugs that interact with warfarin.

ANTIPLATELET DRUGS

1. Acetylsalicylic Acid (ASA, Aspirin)

Actions

Inhibits platelet aggregation by irreversibly inactivating cyclooxygenase, the enzyme responsible for synthesis of the prostaglandin-like substance thromboxane A_2 in platelets (Figure 15–3). Thromboxane A_2 promotes platelet aggregation.

Effects last for the lifetime of the platelet (7 to 10 days).

Uses

Given to reduce the risk of recurrent transient ischemic attacks (TIAs) or stroke in patients who have had transient ischemia of the brain due to fibrin platelet emboli.

Used to decrease the adhesive properties of platelets in patients with diseased arteries, artificial blood vessel shunts and heart valves, and in patients with spontaneous aggregation syndromes.

Administered in the prophylaxis of venous thromboembolism after total hip replacement.

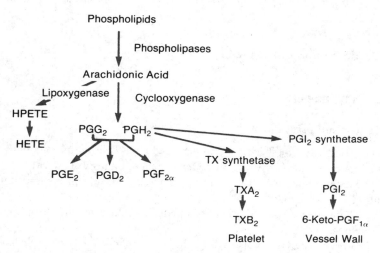

Figure 15–3 Conversion of arachidonic acid to prostaglandins. PG = prostaglandin; TX = thromboxane; H PETE = 12-L-hydroperoxy-5, 8, 10, 14, -eicosatetraenoic acid; HETE = 12-L-hydroxy-5, 8, 10, 14 -eicosatetraenoic acid. (After Mustard JF. Prostaglandins in disease: modification by acetylsalicylic acid. In: Barnett HJM, Hirsh J, Mustard JF, eds. Acetylsalicylic acid, new uses for an old drug. New York: Raven Press, 1982:1.)

Taken to reduce the risk of morbidity and death in patients who have suffered a myocardial infarction.

Adverse Effects

Consult Chapter 25.

2. Sulfinpyrazone

Actions

Competitive inhibitor of cyclooxygenase.

Inhibits platelet adherence and the release reaction. In the release reaction, platelets change shape and undergo a complex secretory process resulting in the release of adenosine disphosphate (ADP) from platelet granules and activation of platelet phospholipase A_2 (see Figure 15–3).

Uses

Used in clinical states in which abnormal platelet behavior is a causative or associated factor (amaurosis fugax [TIAs], thromboembolism associated with vascular and cardiac prostheses, recurrent venous thrombosis, and arteriovenous shunt thrombosis).

Approved for prophylactic use after myocardial infarction.

Adverse Effects

Gastric disturbances, skin rashes.

3. Dipyridamole

Actions and Uses

Decreases platelet adhesiveness to damaged endothelium. Inhibits phosphodiesterase and increases cyclic adenosine monophosphate (cAMP).

May also potentiate the effect of prostacyclin (PGI_2), which stimulates platelet adenyl cyclase.

These effects would prevent both platelet aggregation and the release reactions.

However, dipyridamole itself neither prevents nor exerts a prophylactic effect on the incidence of death following myocardial infarction.

A beneficial effect may occur in combination with aspirin or when it is combined prophylactically with warfarin in patients with artificial heart valves.

Adverse Effects

Headache, flushing, dizziness, weakness or syncope, skin rash, gastric irritation, abdominal cramping, emesis.

4. Ticlopidine

Actions

Causes a time- and dose-dependent inhibition of platelet aggregation and release of platelet factors, as well as a prolongation of bleeding time.

Uses

Used to reduce the risk of first or recurrent stroke for patients who have experienced at least one of the following events: complete thromboembolic stroke, minor stroke, reversible ischemic neurological deficit, or transient ischemic attack including transient monocular blindness.

Adverse Effects

Diarrhea, nausea. Diarrhea and gastrointestinal (GI) pain are most frequent.
   Neutropenia has occurred in approximately 2% of patients.
   Bleeding time is prolonged.

FIBRINOLYTIC DRUGS

1. Streptokinase

Actions

Activates plasminogen-plasmin system, giving rise to increased amounts of plasmin, which lyses fibrin clots (Figure 15–4).

Uses

Used to treat pulmonary embolism, deep vein thrombosis and embolism, arteriovenous cannula occlusion, and coronary artery thrombosis.

Adverse Effects

Hemorrhage. Aminocaproic acid is an antidote.
   Because streptokinase depletes the blood of its normal store of plasminogen, spontaneous thrombosis can occur after the effects of streptokinase disappear. To prevent secondary clot formation, heparin should be

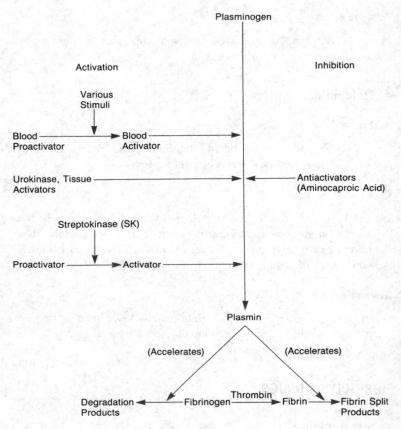

Figure 15–4 Schematic representation of the fibrinolytic system. (After O'Reilly RA. Drugs used in disorders of coagulation. In: Katzung BG, ed. Basic and clinical pharmacology. 5th ed. Appleton & Lange, Norwalk: 1992:466.)

given immediately after the effects of streptokinase cease, followed by oral anticoagulants for 7 days.

2. Urokinase

Action

Converts plasminogen to plasmin.

Uses

Treatment of pulmonary embolism and coronary artery thrombosis.

Adverse Effects

Hemorrhage. Discontinue if there is bleeding and administer fresh whole blood or fresh-frozen plasma. If these measures fail, the use of aminocaproic acid is suggested.

3. Alteplase (Tissue Plasminogen Activator [TPA])

Actions

Binds to fibrin in a thrombus and converts the entrapped plasminogen to plasmin.

The clot selectivity of TPA enables it to lyse clots without having a significant effect on circulating plasminogen.

Has a half-life of about 5 minutes, compared to about 23 minutes for streptokinase.

Uses

Lysis of suspected occlusive coronary artery thrombi associated with evolving transmural myocardial infarction.

Reduces mortality associated with acute myocardial infarction (AMI). Improves ventricular function following AMI and reduces incidence of congestive heart failure.

Adverse Effects

Hemorrhage.

FIBRINOLYTIC INHIBITORS: HEMOSTATIC AGENTS

1. Aminocaproic Acid

Actions

Inhibits fibrinolysis by competitively inhibiting the binding of plasminogen and plasmin to fibrin.

Uses

To treat excessive bleeding resulting from systemic hyperfibrinolysis and urinary fibrinolysis.

As an adjunct in replacement therapy in hemophiliac patients undergoing tooth extraction.

Adverse Effects

Nausea, diarrhea, vomiting.

2. Aprotinin

Actions

Potent proteinase inhibitor, extracted from bovine lung tissue that has an inhibitory action on plasmin activator. Also directly inhibits plasmin.

Uses

To treat patients with conditions caused by excessive fibrinolysis, which occur during surgery (including open heart surgery and prosthetic surgery), and pathologic obstetrical bleeding conditions, such as abruptio placentae.

Adverse Effects

Allergic reactions (such as flushing, tachycardia, itching, rash, and urticaria), dyspnea, sweating, palpitations, nausea.

VITAMIN K₁, VITAMIN K₂, AND MENADIONE

Actions

Vitamin K is not a single chemical but a collection of structurally-related substances that stimulate the hepatic synthesis of vitamin K–dependent clotting factors. Collectively, they are often referred to simply as vitamin K.

Vitamin K_1 (phytonadione) and vitamin K_2 (menaquinone) are found in plant leaves and vegetable oils and are synthesized in large quantities by bacteria in the intestinal tract. Vitamins K_1 and K_2 are well absorbed from the GI tract if bile salts are present. Vitamin K_1 is also formulated for subcutaneous absorption.

Menadione (vitamin K_3) is a synthetic chemical that does not require bile for absorption. It is also available as a water-soluble salt, menadione sodium bisulfite, for parenteral administration.

Menadiol tetrasodium diphosphate is another water-soluble salt of menadione, intended for oral or parenteral administration.

Uses

To treat a deficiency resulting from the inadequate intake, absorption, or utilization of vitamin K.

To antagonize the actions of oral anticoagulants.

To treat newborns who have only 20 to 40% of adult levels of prothrombin. For the prophylaxis and treatment of hemorrhagic diseases of the newborn, the water-soluble vitamin K analogues are not as safe as phytonadione.

To reverse the hypoprothrombinemia resulting from the actions of broad-spectrum antibiotics, which can kill vitamin K-producing bacteria in the colon.

Adverse Effects

Temporary refractoriness to oral anticoagulant therapy.

An overdose of vitamin K in an infant can produce hemolytic anemia or kernicterus.

Drugs and the Thyroid

Function of the Thyroid Gland

The thyroid synthesizes, stores, and secretes L-triiodothyronine (T_3) and
L-thyroxine (T_4).

To do this, the thyroid

- actively extracts iodide from the plasma, and
- oxidizes it to iodine before coupling the iodine to the amino acid tyrosine, forming either monoiodotyrosine or diiodotyrosine. T_3 is formed from one molecule each of monoiodotyrosine and diiodotyrosine. T_4 is produced from two molecules of diiodotyrosine.

Once synthesized, T_3 and T_4 are

- stored within the gland as thyroglobulin, and
- released into the circulation following stimulation of the gland by the thyroid-stimulating hormone (TSH). Some of the T_4 released is subsequently converted to T_3.

The activity of the thyroid gland is controlled by

- the release of hypothalamic thyrotropic-releasing hormone, which in turn
- stimulates the secretion of pituitary TSH. TSH increases the synthesis and secretion of T_3 and T_4.

A balance exists between secretion of TSH and the levels of T_3 and T_4.

- An increase in plasma T_3 and T_4 decreases TSH secretion.
- A decrease in plasma T_3 and T_4 increases TSH secretion.

Once secreted, T_3 and T_4 are highly bound to specific plasma proteins called thyroid-binding globulin and thyroid-binding prealbumin. Only T_3 and T_4 not bound to these plasma proteins (free T_3 and T_4) enter body cells to exert an effect. T_3 produces a more rapid effect than T_4 because it is less bound to plasma proteins. Figure 16–1 presents the principal features of the biosynthesis and metabolism of thyroid hormones.

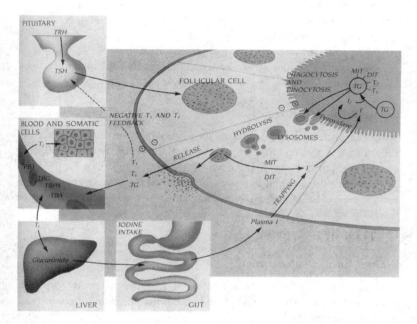

Figure 16–1 Principal features of the biosynthesis and metabolism of thyroid hormones. (After Schimmer BP, George SR. Thyroid Hormones and Antithyroid Drugs. In: Kalant H, Roschlau W, eds. Principles of Medical Pharmacology. 5th ed. Toronto: BC Decker, 1989:444–450.)

Actions of T_3 And T_4

High-affinity binding sites for T_3 and T_4 exist in the nucleus, mitochondria, and plasma membranes of the hormone-responsive tissues (pituitary, liver, kidney, heart, skeletal muscle, lung, and intestine). T_4 receptor affinity is 10 times lower than T_3 affinity.

T_3 and T_4 increase tissue metabolic rate and mitochondrial protein synthesis. They also stimulate the cell membrane sodium pump. T_3 and T_4 are necessary for the maturation and development of the central nervous and skeletal systems. Thyroid deficiency in childhood results in cretinism, a condition characterized by growth failure and mental retardation.

HYPOTHYROIDISM

Hypothyroidism is characterized by low circulating levels of T_3 and T_4, or rarely, tissue resistance to the thyroid hormones. Hypothyroidism can result from pathology in

- the thyroid (primary hypothyroidism),
- the pituitary (secondary hypothyroidism),
- the hypothalamus (tertiary hypothyroidism), and
- the peripheral tissues (generalized resistance to thyroid hormones, usually caused by a defect in the beta receptor for T_4 and T_3).

Symptoms of Hypothyroidism

Symptoms include fatigue, swelling of the hands and around the eyes, constipation, dry skin, and menstrual irregularities. When hypothyroidism is severe, the patient may have a guttural voice, thickened boggy skin (myxedema), slow mental processes, loss of body hair, intolerance to cold, ascites, pericardial effusion, coma, and death.

Drugs for Hypothyroidism

L-Thyroxine (Levothyroxine)

Oral and injectable forms of L-thyroxine (T_4) are the preferred treatment. Converted in part to T_3 in the body, T_4 provides a reliable source of both thyroid hormones.

L-Triiodothyronine (Liothyronine)

Liothyronine (T_3) is 2.5 to 3.3 times more potent than T_4 and its effects are seen sooner. However, stabilization of a patient on T_3 may be more difficult because it is cleared faster than T_4. Treatment with T_4 provides a reliable source of both T_3 and T_4.

Adverse Effects

An overdosage of either T_3 or T_4 can induce hyperthyroidism (eg, heat intolerance, weakness, fatigue, nervousness, insomnia, and tachycardia). For drug interactions with T_3 and T_4 consult an appropriate reference source.

HYPERTHYROIDISM

Hyperthyroidism is a syndrome characterized by excessive production and release of T_3 and T_4. The more common causes of hyperthyroidism are:

- Graves' disease (the most common cause of hyperthyroidism) — caused by the production of an antibody capable of stimulating the thyrotrophin (TSH) receptor on the surface of the thyroid cells
- Toxic adenoma — a benign tumor of the thyroid capable of producing excessive amounts of thyroid hormones

- Toxic multinodular goitre (found primarily in the elderly) — a condition in which thyroid follicles autonomously produce excessive quantities of T_3 and T_4
- Subacute thyroiditis — results from the excessive release of T_3 and T_4 from an inflamed thyroid gland

Symptoms of Hyperthyroidism

These include heat intolerance, bruit over the thyroid, a hyperkinetic circulatory state (including a rapid heart rate and dysrhythmias), and dyspnea. Unusual muscle fatigue, irritability, and the presence of eye signs, such as lid lag, weakness of the extraocular muscle, and proptosis may also be seen.

Thyroid Storm

Thyroid storm is a rare medical emergency. It is characterized by thyrotoxicosis, with fever, tachycardia or tachyarrhythmias, and altered mental state. Thyroid storm must be treated aggressively because its mortality is high. Treatment includes

- high doses of propylthiouracil (PTU) or methimazole (MMI),
- IV sodium iodide or oral strong iodine solution,
- beta blockers,
- glucocorticoids, and
- measures to ensure that hyperpyrexia, congestive heart failure, cardiac arrhythmias, and dehydration are properly managed.

Drugs for Hyperthyroidism

1. Propylthiouracil and Methimazole

Actions

PTU and MMI prevent the formation of T_3 and T_4, by blocking the oxidative iodination of tyrosine. PTU also impairs the peripheral conversion of T_4 to T_3.

Uses

PTU and MMI are used to prepare patients for thyroid surgery, to assist in the management of patients in thyrotoxic crisis, and to treat chronic hyperthyroidism. Several weeks to months of treatment with PTU or MMI restores euthyroidism in Graves' patients.

Adverse Effects

Important adverse effects include GI upset, mild elevation in liver enzymes, and rash. Rare, but more serious, adverse effects include liver toxicity and agranulocytosis.

Care must be taken in prescribing PTU or MMI during pregnancy because these drugs cross the placenta and can cause fetal goitre and hypothyroidism. PTU is frequently preferred because of the unresolved contention that MMI may cause the rare congenital complication, aplasia cutis.

Both PTU and MMI are contraindicated in nursing mothers.

2. Potassium Iodide, Sodium Iodide, and Strong Iodine Solution

Actions

Large doses of these drugs inhibit, at least temporarily, organic iodine formation and the production and release of T_3 and T_4. High doses may also prevent the effects of TSH.

Uses

These products are used to prepare hyperthyroid patients for thyroidectomy.

Intravenous sodium iodide or oral strong iodine solution may also be used with PTU or MMI to treat thyroid storm.

Adverse Effects

Unpleasant taste, burning of mouth, sore mouth and throat, hypersalivation, painful sialadenitis, acne and other rashes, productive cough, angioedema with swelling of the larynx, dyspnea in sensitive individuals.

3. Beta Blockers (see Chapter 6)

Actions

Beta blockers are important adjuvant drugs because they reduce hyperthyroid symptoms caused by excessive beta adrenergic stimulation (eg, palpitations, tremor, and sweating). Beta blockers generally do not alter T_4 levels. However, nonselective beta blockers, such as propranolol, may decrease circulating T_3 levels.

Drugs for the Treatment of Diabetes Mellitus

DIABETES MELLITUS

- Diabetes mellitus is a chronic metabolic disturbance that is characterized by fasting or postprandial hyperglycemia.
- Diabetes mellitus is not a single entity. It is a heterogeneous syndrome caused by an absolute or relative lack of insulin, resistance to the action of insulin, or both.
- When severe, diabetes mellitus affects carbohydrate, lipid, and protein metabolism.
- Severe long-term diabetes mellitus may lead to complications involving small blood vessels (microangiopathy), large blood vessels (macroangiopathy), and nerve damage (neuropathy) that affect multiple organs and systems.

DIAGNOSIS OF DIABETES MELLITUS

The diagnosis of diabetes mellitus is established by any of the following:

- The presence of symptoms of diabetes plus a casual (random) plasma glucose level ≥ 11.1 mmol/L.
- A fasting plasma glucose level ≥ 7.0 mmol/L. This must be confirmed by a second test on a subsequent day.
- A plasma glucose level ≥ 11.1 mmol/L at 2 hours after a 75 g oral glucose tolerance test.

GOALS OF THERAPY

To maintain the long-term health of the person affected with diabetes, therapy should

- Control symptoms
- Establish and maintain optimum metabolic control, while avoiding hypoglycemia
- Prevent, or minimize the risk of, complications
- Achieve optimum control of comorbidities such as hypertension or dyslipidemia

CLASSIFICATION OF DIABETES MELLITUS

- **Type 1 diabetes mellitus** (insulin-dependent diabetes mellitus, IDDM) is due to beta cell destruction, usually leading to absolute insulin deficiency – **treated with insulin**.
- **Type 2 diabetes mellitus** (non–insulin-dependent diabetes mellitus, NIDDM) ranges from predominant insulin resistance, with relative insulin deficiency, to predominant insulin secretory defect, with insulin resistance – **treated with oral agents and/or insulin**.
- **Gestational diabetes mellitus** is defined as onset or recognition of glucose intolerance in pregnancy – **treated with insulin**.
- **Other specific types,** including the genetic syndrome MODY (maturity-onset diabetes of youth), other genetic syndromes associated with diabetes, pancreatic disease, infectious agents, other diseases leading to carbohydrate intolerance, and drug-induced carbohydrate intolerance.

TARGETS FOR CONTROL

- **Control of blood glucose** reduces the risk of long-term complications in type 1 and type 2 diabetes; however, euglycemia is difficult to attain and maintain. The main risk of tight control of blood glucose levels is the increased risk of hypoglycemic episodes. Frequent hypoglycemia may lead to hypoglycemia unawareness.
- **Control of serum lipids** reduces the risk of cardiovascular events, which are the main cause of morbidity and mortality in diabetes. Diabetes over age 30 is considered a very high risk for coronary artery disease. Therapy includes statins for elevated LDL-cholesterol and fibrates for elevated triglyceride and/or low HDL-cholesterol (see Chapter 14).
- **Control of blood pressure** (below 130/85 mm Hg) is an additional goal of therapy. Diabetes, particularly type 2, is frequently associated with hypertension.

NON-DRUG TREATMENT OF TYPES 1 AND 2 DIABETES MELLITUS

Nonpharmacologic therapy plays a pivotal role in the treatment of types 1 and 2 diabetes.

- Type 1 diabetes must receive insulin immediately, along with non-drug therapy.
- In the absence of symptoms, type 2 diabetics usually receive nonpharmacologic therapy as the first step in treating the disease. Drug therapy is instituted in type 2 asymptomatic diabetes only if nonpharmacologic therapy fails to establish euglycemia.
- Non-drug therapy can be found in standard texts on diabetes management. It includes:
  - ♦ Education, to make the patient a full participant in the diabetes health care team
  - ♦ Nutritional management, designed to individualize the diet
  - ♦ Instruction in self-monitoring of glucose levels
  - ♦ A program of physical activity
  - ♦ Periodic reassessments to detect comorbidities and complications

DRUG TREATMENT OF TYPE 1 DIABETES MELLITUS

Insulin

- Type 1 patients have little or no insulin in the pancreas.
- These people usually experience an abrupt onset of symptoms, insulin deficiency, and dependence on injected insulin to sustain life.
- Human insulin should be started at the time of diagnosis. Table 17–1 presents commonly used human insulin preparations. For optimum

Table 17–1
Human Insulin and Analogues

Type of Insulin	Onset (h)	Peak (h)	Duration (h)
Rapid-acting insulin lispro	0.5 – 0.75	0.75 – 2.5	3.5 – 4.75
Short-acting regular insulin	0.5 – 1	0.75 – 4.5	5.0 – 7.5
Intermediate-acting NPH	1 – 2	4 – 12	12 – 24
Intermediate-acting Lente	2 – 4	7 – 15	12 – 24
Long-acting Ultralente	3 – 4	8 – 16	24 – 28

NPH = neutral protamine Hagedorn.
(After Boctor MA. Diabetes Mellitus. In: [editor's names] eds. Therapeutic Choices. 3rd ed. Ottawa: Canadian Pharmacist Association, 2000:613–628.)

control, regular insulin should be administered 20 to 30 minutes before meals. Rapid-acting insulin may be more conveniently administered shortly before eating.

Insulin Regimens For Type 1 Diabetics (Table 17–2)

Intensive treatment regimens control blood glucose more effectively than conventional regimens and reduce the risk of long-term diabetic complications. Newly diagnosed type 1 diabetics, as well as type 1 diabetes who

Table 17–2
Insulin Regimens

	Rapid or Short-Acting Insulin	Intermediate or Long-Acting Insulins	Remarks
Conventional	None	Once daily NPH or Lente before breakfast	Unlikely to achieve control
	None	Twice daily NPH or Lente at breakfast and supper	Improved morning levels
	Regular or insulin lispro at breakfast and supper	NPH or Lente at breakfast and supper	Most widely used regimen; better meal control
	Regular or insulin lispro at breakfast and supper	NPH or Lente at breakfast, Ultralente at supper	Ultralente more likely to last until next morning
	Regular or insulin lispro at breakfast and supper	NPH or Lente at breakfast, NPH or Lente at bedtime	More likely to last until next morning
Intensive Multidose Insulin Regimen (MDI)	Regular or insulin lispro before each meal	NPH, Lente, or Ultra lente at supper or bedtime	Usually good control, flexible
	Regular or insulin lispro before each meal	NPH, Lente or Ultra lente twice daily at breakfast and supper or bedtime	Better suited for people with varying schedules
Intensive continuous subcutaneous insulin injection	Regular or insulin lispro basal and boluses as per program	None	Most flexible, can achieve even better control than MDI; most expensive; diabetic keto-acidosis may occur quickly with discontinuation

NPH = neutral protamine Hagedorn.
(After Boctor MA. Diabetes Mellitus. In: Gray J. eds. Therapeutic Choices. 3rd ed. Ottawa: Canadian Pharmacists Association, 2000:613–628.)

have not achieved control on conventional therapy, should be offered an intensive diabetes management option.

Adverse Effects of Insulin Therapy

Hypoglycemia is the most common adverse effect of insulin and occurs most frequently in patients on tight diabetic control.

- **Mild hypoglycemia** is manifested by adrenergic symptoms, such as sweating, tremors, tachycardia, hunger, and general weakness. Treat with an oral source of sugar.
- **Severe hypoglycemia** requires assistance in its recognition and/or treatment. Neuroglycopenic symptoms, including confusion, altered behavior, and disorientation, can progress to seizures and coma, and prevent the patient from treating the episode. If the patient is conscious, an oral glucose preparation should be used. In unconscious patients, intramuscular or subcutaneous glucagon temporarily increases blood glucose allowing for the intake of oral carbohydrate. Glucagon is not effective in malnourished patients, or alcohol-induced hypoglycemia. Intravenous dextrose is the treatment of choice under these circumstances.

Localized fat hypertrophy is most often the result of frequent reutilization of the same injection site.

Allergic reactions such as urticaria, angioedema rashes, and local erythema, are rare with human insulin.

Immune-mediated insulin resistance, due to production of anti-insulin antibodies, is rare with human insulin.

DRUG TREATMENT OF TYPE 2 DIABETES MELLITUS

All drugs presented below are used as adjuncts to diet and exercise in asymptomatic type 2 diabetic patients whose diabetes cannot be controlled satisfactorily by diet alone.

Drug treatment is warranted initially in symptomatic type 2 patients.

1. Drugs That Increase the Secretion of Insulin

A. Sulfonylureas (Acetohexamide, Chlorpropamide, Gliclazide, Glyburide, Tolbutamide)

Actions

Sulfonylureas require the presence of insulin to be effective. They

1. stimulate the pancreatic release of insulin,
2. increase the action of insulin on the liver to decrease hepatic gluconeogenesis, and

3. increase glucose utilization (Figure 17–1).

Adverse Effects

Severe hypoglycemia, nausea, epigastric fullness, heartburn, and allergic skin reactions, such as pruritus, erythema, urticaria, and morbiliform or maculopapular eruptions. For a list of the many drug interactions with sulfonylureas, consult a reference text.

B. Repaglinide

Actions

Repaglinide lowers blood glucose by stimulating the release of insulin. Repaglinide is a short-acting drug, which is effective in regulating meal-

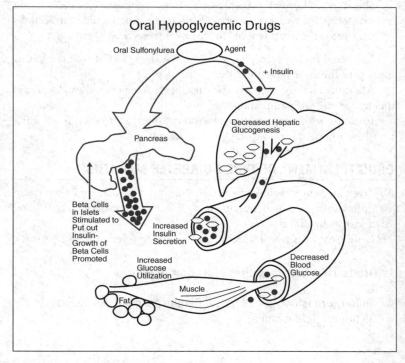

Figure 17–1 Suggested actions of sulfonylurea drugs. (After Waife SO. Oral hypoglycemic agents. In: Diabetes Mellitus. Indianapolis: Eli Lilly, 1980:123.)

related glucose loads. Because of its short action, repaglinide should only be taken with meals.

Adverse Effects

Hypoglycemia, especially if the meal is not taken, and weight gain.

2. Drugs that Increase Tissue Sensitivity to Insulin

A. Metformin

Actions

Metformin requires the presence of insulin to lower blood glucose. Metformin appears to increase the action of insulin in peripheral tissues but its primary action is to reduce hepatic glucose output by inhibiting gluconeogenesis. It may also decrease plasma glucose by reducing the absorption of glucose from the intestine. Used alone, metformin does not cause hypoglycemia, but it can potentiate the hypoglycemic effects of insulin and sulfonylureas.

Adverse Effects

Metallic taste in the mouth, epigastric discomfort, nausea, and vomiting. For a list of the drug interactions with metformin consult a reference text.

B. Thiazolidinediones (Pioglitazone and Rosiglitazone)

Actions

Thiazolidinediones improve sensitivity to insulin in muscle and adipose tissue and inhibit hepatic gluconeogenesis. By decreasing insulin resistance, thiazolidinediones improve glucose control, decrease hepatic glucose output, increase insulin-dependent glucose disposal in skeletal muscle, and reduce circulating insulin levels. These drugs are used alone to treat type 2 diabetes, in patients not controlled by exercise and diet. Thiazolidinediones are also used in combination with metformin and/or sulfonylureas, in type 2 diabetics who were not controlled with the original therapy.

Adverse Effects

Weight gain due to subcutaneous fat increases, and occasionally, water retention.

3. Drugs that Delay the Digestion of Complex Carbohydrates (Acarbose)

Actions

Acarbose inhibits alpha-glucosidase in the brush border of the small intestine. Alpha-glucosidase is responsible for the hydrolysis of sucrose into absorbable monosaccharides. By inhibiting this enzyme, acarbose delays glucose absorption, reduces postprandial hyperglycemia, and decreases glycosylated hemoglobin (HbA_{1C}) in type 2 diabetes mellitus patients.

Adverse Effects

Flatulence, diarrhea, and abdominal pain.

4. Insulin

Insulin may be used alone in type 2 diabetics. It may also be used in combination with an oral agent in a nighttime insulin/daytime pill regimen. Because of their underlying resistance to insulin, many type 2 diabetics require higher doses of insulin.

18

Adrenal Corticosteroids

HORMONES SECRETED BY THE ADRENAL CORTEX

1. Glucocorticoids
2. Mineralocorticoids
3. Sex hormones (discussed in Chapter 19)

GLUCOCORTICOIDS

Synthesis and Secretion of Cortiosol (Figure 18–1)

Cortisol (hydrocortisone) is the major endogenous glucocorticoid. It is synthesized in, and secreted from, the adrenal cortex in response to the release of adrenocorticotropic hormone (ACTH) from the pituitary. ACTH secretion is controlled by the release of corticotropin-releasing factor (CRF) from the hypothalamus. High levels of glucocorticoids suppress CRF secretion, thereby reducing ACTH release, and preventing cortisol secretion.

Mechanism of Action of Glucocorticoids (Figure 18–2 and Table 18–1)

Tissue selectivity for glucocorticoids depends on the presence of specific corticosteroid receptors in the cytoplasm of the target cell. Glucocorticoids pass from the blood into the cell and combine with the receptor. The receptor-steroid complex then moves into the nucleus where it stimulates new transcription of both messenger ribonucleic acid (mRNA) and (ribosomal) rRNA, a process essential to the physiologic/pharmacologic effects of the glucocorticoids.

Metabolic Actions of Glucocorticoids (Figure 18–3)

1. Impair glucose utilization, while increasing its synthesis. Blood sugar levels rise.

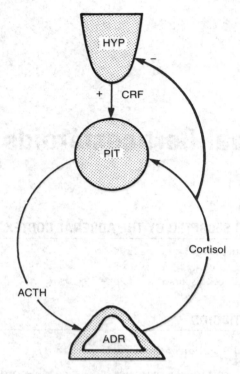

Figure 18–1 Diagrammatic representation of hypothalamic-pituitary-adrenal axis. Pituitary adrenocorticotropic hormone (ACTH) secretion is regulated by negative feedback effects of cortisol on the pituitary. Hypothalamic drive of ACTH release is mediated by corticotrophin-releasing factor (CRF). Cortisol inhibits pituitary response to CRF and may also inhibit the secretion of CRF. (After Reichlin S. Current concepts of neural control of the pituitary gland: normal physiology and pathologic implications. Kalamazoo, (MI): Scope publications, The Upjohn Co, 1978:33.)

2. Stimulate fat and muscle catabolism, releasing FFA, glycerol, and amino acids, increasing their levels in blood.
3. Increase gluconeogenesis.
4. Increase glucagon secretion, further accelerating hepatic glucose output.
5. Indirectly stimulate insulin release by increasing blood sugar. Direct steroid actions on fat are counterbalanced, in part, by the effects of insulin, which stimulates lipogenesis and inhibits lipolysis. The result is a redistribution of fat. At sites where the actions of corticosteroids predominate, fat is lost; in areas where insulin dominates, fat accumulates.
6. Reduce calcium absorption (by blocking actions of vitamin D) and increase calcium renal clearance. These actions can result in osteoporosis.

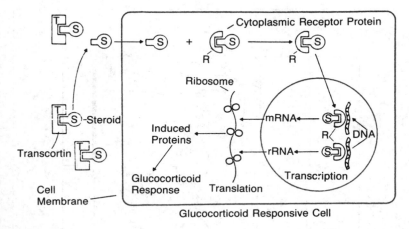

Glucocorticoid Responsive Cell

Figure 18–2 Schematic representation of the mechanism of action of glucocorticoids.mRNA = messenger ribonucleic acid; rRNA = ribosomal ribonucleicacid; DNA = deoxyribonucleic acid (After Swartz SL, Dluhy RG. Corticosteroids. Clinical pharmacology and therapeutic use. Drugs 1978; 16:243.)

Anti-inflammatory and Immunosuppressive Action of Glucocorticoids

1. Potentiate vasoconstrictor effects of epinephrine and norepinephrine, reducing blood flow, redness, and heat.
2. Decrease capillary permeability, reducing plasma loss into inflamed tissues, which decreases swelling.
3. Decrease mast cell accumulation at the site of inflammation, reducing histamine release.
4. Reduce prostaglandin E_2 (PGE_2) synthesis, decreasing the pain-producing actions of histamine and bradykinin.
5. Reduce neutrophil migration to the inflammatory site(s).
6. Decrease T-lymphocyte levels in blood, reducing cell-mediated immunity.

Table 18–1
Presence of Glucocorticoid Receptors in Tissues

Tissues with Specific Glucocorticoid Receptors			Tissues with No Detectable, or Low Glucocorticoid Receptors		
Brain	Heart	Liver	Bladder	Prostate	Steroid-resistant
Lymphoid	Retina	Smooth	Steroid-	Seminal	lymphoid cells
tissue	Fibroblasts	muscle	resistant	vesicle	Uterus
Testes	Lung	Intestine	fibroblasts		
Kidney		Skeletal			
Stomach		muscle			

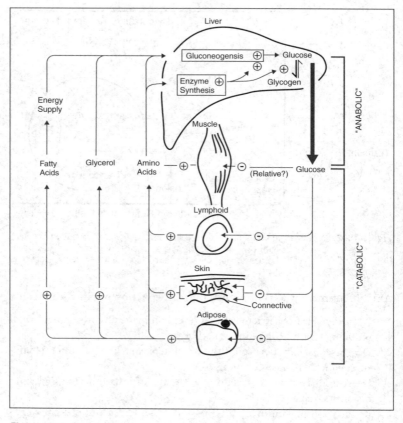

Figure 18–3 Glucocorticoid action on carbohydrate, lipid and protein metabolism. Arrows indicate the general flow of substrates in response to the catabolic and anabolic actions of the glucocorticoids when unopposed by secondary secretions of other hormones. + and – signs indicate stimulation and inhibition, respectively. (After Baxter JD, Forsham PH. Tissue effects of glucocorticoids. Am J Med 1972; 53:573–589.)

7. Reduce fibrin deposition, capillary fibroblast proliferation, deposition of collagen, and cicatrization.

Adverse Effects of Glucocorticoids

1. Musculoskeletal — myopathy, osteoporosis, fractures.
2. GI — peptic ulceration, hemorrhage, perforation, pancreatitis.
3. CNS — psychiatric disorders.
4. Eye — glaucoma, cataracts.
5. Cardiovascular and renal — hypertension, Na^+ and water retention, hypokalemic alkalosis.

6. Metabolic — precipitation of genetic diabetes mellitus, hyperosmolar nonketotic coma, hyperlipidemia, centripetal obesity.
7. Endocrine — growth failure, secondary amenorrhea, suppression of hypothalamic-pituitary-adrenal system.
8. Inhibition of fibroblasts — impaired wound healing, subcutaneous tissue atrophy.
9. Suppression of immune response — superinfections.

SYNTHETIC GLUCOCORTICOIDS

Rationale Behind Synthetic Glucocorticoids (Table 18–2)

Cortisol possesses both significant glucocorticoid and mineralocorticoid actions. Synthetic glucocorticoids have been synthesized with the aim of accentuating glucocorticoid activity and reducing or abolishing mineralocorticoid properties. The anti-inflammatory effects of the various corticosteroids correlate with their relative glucocorticoid potencies. Because synthetic corticosteroids are more potent glucocorticoids than cortisone and cortisol (hydrocortisone), they are used in lower doses. Synthetic glu-

Table 18–2
Comparison of Corticosteroids

Drug	Anti-Inflammatory Potency*	Equivalent Potency* (mg)	Sodium Retaining Potency	Biologic Half-Life (h)
Cortisol [A]	1	20	2+	8–12
Cortisone [A]	0.8	25	2+	8–12
Prednisone [B]	3.5	5	1+	18–36
Prednisolone [B]	4	5	1+	18–36
Methylprednisolone [B]	5	4	0	18–36
Triamcinolone [B]	5	4	0	18–36
Paramethasone [C]	10	2	0	36–54
Betamethasone [C]	25	0.6	0	36–54
Dexamethasone [C]	30	0.75	0	36–54

*Potency is defined as mg for mg equivalence with cortisol.
[A] – Short-acting corticosteroids; [B] – Intermediate-acting corticosteroids; [C] – Long-acting corticosteroids
(Modified from Swartz SL, Dluhy RG. Corticosteroids. Clinical pharmacology and therapeutic use. Drugs 1978; 16:238–255.)

cocorticoids also have longer half-lives than either cortisol or cortisone and are given less frequently.

THERAPEUTIC USES FOR GLUCOCORTICOIDS

Replacement Therapy

Primary Adrenal Insufficiency

Both glucocorticoids and mineralocorticoids are administered in primary adrenal insufficiency (Addison's Disease) because patients are deficient in both cortisol and aldosterone.

Secondary Adrenal Insufficiency

Adrenal insufficiency secondary to pituitary insufficiency is characterized by low levels of cortisol. Aldosterone secretion is normal. Cortisol can be given daily with two-thirds of the dose in the morning and one-third around 4 pm.

Congenital Adrenal Hyperplasia (Adrenogenital Syndrome)

This condition results from adrenal cortical enzyme deficiencies in the synthesis of cortisol. As a result of lower cortisol levels, ACTH secretion is increased, elevating the synthesis and secretion of adrenal androgens. Evidence of the condition in the female is often seen at birth as masculinization of the external genitalia. Diagnosis of the adrenal genital syndrome in males may not be made until later in infancy or in childhood. Treatment involves administration of a glucocorticoid to suppress ACTH secretion. It may also be necessary to administer a mineralocorticoid if a reduction in both glucocorticoid and mineralocorticoid synthesis occurs. It is advisable to give a larger dose of the glucocorticoid at bedtime to suppress the normal peak secretion of ACTH during the night.

Suppressive Therapy

Dosage Protocols

Short-term, high-dose is used for the treatment of emergencies, such as status asthmaticus and anaphylactic shock. This type of protocol has the least likelihood of adverse effects.

Long-term, low-dose is often appropriate for many diseases, such as asthma or arthritis.

Long-term, high-dose is often required for severe conditions such as autoimmune hemolytic anemia and temporal arteritis. This type of regimen is most likely to cause adverse effects.

Alternate-day therapy is intended to minimize the consequences of chronic glucocorticoid treatment. Start the patient on a daily dose until relief is obtained. Then convert gradually to alternate-day treatment by doubling the daily dose and administering it as a single dose on alternate mornings. Use intermediate-acting steroids, such as prednisone, so that treatment is effective for about 1.5 days, but still allows 0.5 days for the pituitary-adrenal responsiveness to return before the next dose.

Uses

Inflammatory diseases of the intestine, bronchioles, nose, eyes, ears, skin and joints.

Allergic diseases — used only in situations not adequately controlled by less dangerous agents, such as antihistamines.

Rheumatic carditis, collagen vascular diseases, renal diseases, liver diseases, and shock.

MINERALOCORTICOIDS

Synthesis and Secretion of Aldosterone

Aldosterone is synthesized in the adrenal cortex. Secretion is increased by stimulation of the renin-angiotensin system. Hyperkalemia increases and hypokalemia decreases aldosterone secretion. During stress, ACTH may stimulate aldosterone secretion. Increased levels of aldosterone are not sustained by prolonged elevated ACTH secretion.

Actions of Mineralocorticoids

Mineralocorticoids increase Na^+ reabsorption and K^+ and H^+ secretion in the distal convoluted tubules and collecting ducts of the kidneys (see Chapter 13).

Adverse Effects of Mineralocorticoids

Mineralocorticoids increase salt and water retention and potassium loss. Their effects include hypertension, edema, hypokalemia, cardiac enlargement, and congestive heart failure.

19

Sex Hormones

ESTROGENS

Naturally Occurring Estrogens

Estradiol — secreted by the ovaries. The estrogen of greatest physiologic significance.
- **Estrone** — also secreted by the ovaries.
- **Estriol** — a metabolic product of both estradiol and estrone.

Control of Estrogen Secretion

In females, follicle stimulating hormone (FSH) stimulates the ovaries to produce ova and estrogens. Luteinizing hormone (LH) acts first, in concert with FSH, to promote ovulation, and later alone to stimulate progesterone and estrogen synthesis by the corpus luteum (Figure 19–1).

Actions

Tissue selectivity of estrogens is achieved by the presence of specific soluble protein receptors found in the cytoplasm of sensitive cells. Estrogens pass from the blood into the cell and combine with these receptors. Following transfer of the receptor-estrogen complex into the nucleus, the estrogen interacts with chromatin to produce the metabolic changes essential for estrogen action. The principle behind the estrogen-receptor interaction is similar to that previously described for corticosteroids (see Figure 18–2).

Estrogens are:

1. Essential for the development of the reproductive organs in the female. They

   - increase mitotic activity and stratification of cells of the vaginal epithelium and cause a proliferation of uterine cervical mucosa,

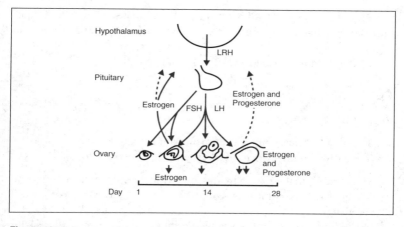

Figure 19–1 Summary of endocrine changes during the menstrual cycle. The dashed arrows indicate inhibitory effects and the sold lines stimulatory effects. (After The gonads: development and function of the reproductive system. In: Ganong WF Review of Medical Physiology. 11th ed. Los Altos: Lange, 1983:336.)

- produce endometrial mitoses,
- increase the height of the epithelium,
- improve blood supply and capillary permeability of uterine vessels,
- increase uterine water and electrolyte content, and
- stimulate stromal development and ductal growth in the breasts.

2. Responsible for the accelerated growth phase in maturing females and for closing the epiphyses of the long bones at puberty.
3. Partially responsible for the maintenance of normal skin and blood vessel structure.
4. Responsible for the decreased rate of bone resorption in females.

Pharmacokinetics

Oral estradiol is rapidly inactivated in the portal circulation during its first pass through the liver. Injecting estradiol as either the benzoate, cypionate, dipropionate, or valerate ester can circumvent this problem. Given this way, estradiol has a long duration of action.

Ethinyl estradiol, mestranol, quinestrol, and diethylstilbestrol (among others) are synthetic estrogens that are not rapidly inactivated by first-pass metabolism.

Conjugated estrogens are a combination of the sodium salts of the sulfate esters of estrogenic substances, principally estrone and equilin. The esters are similar to the type excreted by pregnant mares. The various preparations contain 50 to 65% estrone sodium sulfate and 20 to 35% equilin sodium sulfate. These products are effective orally, parenterally, and vaginally.

17-β-Estradiol is also formulated as a skin patch.

Uses

Replacement Therapy

1. Treatment of the symptoms of menopause.
2. Prevention and treatment of postmenopausal osteoporosis.

- Concern that estrogen treatment may increase the risk of breast and uterine carcinoma has stopped many women from taking these drugs.
- Estrogen treatment can cause uterine bleeding, increase the risk for venous thromboembolic events, produce cholelithiasis, cause headaches, and result in pain and enlargement of the breasts.
- Many women prefer other drugs such as the bisphosphonates for the prevention and treatment of postmenopausal osteoporosis. Bisphosphonates, such as etidronate and alendronate, inhibit osteoclast-mediated bone resorption and are not encumbered by the toxicities of estrogens or the concerns that estrogen therapy may increase the risk of breast or uterine cancer.
- The selective estrogen receptor modulator, raloxifene (see below), is also effective in preventing postmenopausal osteoporosis.

3. Used in conditions where the ovaries fail to develop:

- In Turner's syndrome, estrogen treatment produces breast enlargement and menses but does not cause the normal growth spurt or ovarian maturation.
- In hypopituitarism replacement therapy in girls, estrogens are administered together with thyroxine and adrenal cortical hormones.

Dysmenorrhea

Estrogens provide relief by inhibiting ovulation. Cyclic therapy with an estrogen-containing oral contraceptive is often successful.

Endometriosis

Estrogen-containing oral contraceptives reduce FSH secretion and provide symptomatic relief in 75 to 100% of cases of endometriosis-associated pain.

Alternatively, the androgen antagonist danazol, which prevents FSH secretion, inhibits ovarian estrogen production, and causes atrophy of endometrial deposits, is used to treat endometriosis-associated pain.

Adverse Effects

Estrogens can produce nausea, vomiting, anorexia, diarrhea, breast tenderness, weight gain due to edema, and hypertension. The effects of estrogens on blood coagulation are discussed under Oral Contraceptives later in this chapter.

ANTIESTROGENS

1. Clomiphene

Actions

Clomiphene competes with estrogens for receptors. By blocking the actions of endogenous estrogens, clomiphene prevents the normal feedback inhibition of FSH and LH secretion. Increased gonadotropin secretion leads to ovarian stimulation, ovulation, and sustained corpus luteum formation.

Uses

Clomiphene is used to treat infertility due to anovulation. It is not effective in women with ovarian or pituitary failure or with undeveloped ovaries.

Adverse Effects

Multiple pregnancy, birth defects, ovarian enlargement, liver dysfunction, hot flashes, abdominal discomfort, visual blurring, spots or flashes, nausea, vomiting, dizziness.

2. Tamoxifen

Actions

Competes with endogenous estrogens for receptors in target tissues, such as breast and uterus. Produces regression of breast cancer in pre- and postmenopausal women.

Uses

Used to treat breast cancer in estrogen receptor–positive tumors.

Adverse Effects

Hot flashes, nausea, vomiting, vaginal bleeding and discharge.

SELECTIVE ESTROGEN RECEPTOR MODULATOR (SERM)

Raloxifene

Actions

Raloxifene acts as an estrogen agonist in the skeleton, to increase bone mineral density in postmenopausal women, and on cholesterol metabolism, to reduce LDL. Raloxifene has estrogen-antagonist effects on breast and uterus. In contrast to estrogens, it does not appear to increase the risk of uterine or breast cancer, or benign breast-related adverse events, such as breast pain, breast enlargement, and fibrocystic disease. Raloxifene does not appear to increase the risk of cardiovascular disease, myocardial infarction, stroke, or any other major arterial cardiovascular event. Raloxifene may increase the risk of venous thrombolytic events.

Uses

Raloxifene is used for the treatment and prevention of osteoporosis in postmenopausal women.

Adverse Effects

Vasodilatation and leg cramps are the most common adverse events.

PROGESTINS

Naturally Occurring Progestin

Progesterone is the naturally occurring progestin. Progesterone is synthesized and secreted by the corpus luteum and placenta (see Figure 19–1).

Actions

Progesterone works in association with estrogens — its effects are only seen in tissues previously stimulated by estrogens.

Both estrogens and progesterone are important in establishing a normal environment for the fertilized egg. Estrogens stimulate growth of sensitive tissue. Progesterone converts newly formed cells into secretory tissue, for example:

- Estrogens increase stromal and ductal development in breasts and progesterone subsequently prepares the glands for lactation.
- Progesterone reduces uterine motility and prepares the estrogen-stimulated endometrium for egg implantation and maintenance of gestation.

Pharmacokinetics

Oral progesterone has little effect because it is rapidly inactivated during the first pass through the liver. Intramuscular (IM) progesterone may be given to circumvent first-pass metabolism. Medroxyprogesterone acetate is a synthetic progestin that can be IM injected or administered orally. Megestrol acetate, norethindrone, norethindrone acetate, and norethynodrel are synthetic progestins that are not rapidly inactivated by first-pass metabolism and can be given orally.

Uses

Progestin therapy is used to treat **dysfunctional uterine bleeding**. This condition often results from endometrial hyperplasia, produced by the continuous action of estradiol together with insufficient progesterone secretion to maintain the endometrium.

Progestin therapy is also used with an estrogen to treat **dysmenorrhea** and **endometriosis**.

Adverse Effects

Possible congenital malformation if administered early in pregnancy, breakthrough bleeding, intercyclic spotting, changes in menstrual flow, amenorrhea, changes in cervical erosion and secretion, breast tenderness, weight gain, and edema.

ORAL CONTRACEPTIVES (OCs)

Types of Products

Oral contraceptives (OCs)contain either a combination of an estrogen plus a progestin, or a progestin alone (Table 19–1).

Safety of Oral Contraceptives

Concern over the safety of OCs has centered on the estrogen component.

- OCs increase the incidence of **venous thromboembolism**. This risk may be reduced significantly by using low-dose estrogen preparations (≤ 50 μg of estrogen).
- The increased risk of MI in women over age 30 appears to be related to estrogen dose. Decreasing the dose of estrogen to 35 μg significantly reduces MI risk. Risk of MI is higher in women > 35 years who smoke.

Table 19–1
Contraceptive Products

Types of Products	Comments

Monophasic oral contraceptives
50 μg estrogen
    EE or mestranol combined with
    ethynodiol, d-norgestrel, or
    norethindrone
< 50 μg estrogen
    35 or 20 μg EE combined with
    desogestrel, ethynodiol acetate,
    LN, norgestimate, NE or NE acetate
	Taken at the same time each day from the 5th to the 26th day of each cycle, all estrogen-containing products suppress ovulation. Bleeding occurs 3 or 4 days after stopping the tablets. Day 1 is the first day of menstruation. Concern over estrogen toxicity has led to low-dose estrogen tablets. Monophasic pills contain the same ratio of estrogen to progestin in each pill

Biphasic oral contraceptives
EE 35 μg/NE 0.5 mg × 10 d;
EE 35 μg/NE 1 mg × 11 d.
Triphasic oral contraceptives
Ratio of estrogen to progestin differs on daily basis between products.
One product contains:
• EE 35 μg/NE 0.5 mg × 7 d;
  EE 35 μg/NE 0.75 mg × 7 d;
  EE 35 μg/NE 1 mg × 7 d.
	The biphasic and triphasic pills provide a dosage pattern that more closely approximates the estrogen-to-progestin ratios that occur during the menstrual cycle. The purpose of introducing the biphasic and triphasic oral contraceptive products is to decrease the incidence and severity of drug-induced adverse effects, such as breakthrough bleeding

Progestin-only products NE	Must be taken every day of the cycle at the same time each day. Inhibits secretion of pituitary gonadotropins, preventing follicular maturation and ovulation, as well as causing changes in cervical mucus and endometrium Somewhat less effective than estrogen-containing products
Injectable products Medroxyprogesterone acetate Levonorgestrel implant	A progestin than is extremely safe and effective. Has prolonged effect. Given every 3 months. Progestin-containing rods are implanted in the subcutaneous tissue of the upper, inner arm. Efficacy close to tubal ligation

Continued

Table 19–1
Contraceptive Products—Continued

Types of Products	Comments
Emergency postcoital contraception	
EE 50 μg/LN 0.25 mg	For both products, the 1st dose should be taken as soon as possible after unprotected intercourse, within 72 hours, followed by a 2nd dose 12 hours later
LN 0.75 mg	

EE = ethinyl estradiol; NE = norethindrone; LN = nevonorgestrel; d = days

ANDROGENS

Naturally Occurring Androgens

Testosterone is the major androgen secreted by the testes. Pituitary LH and FSH stimulate testosterone synthesis and secretion. The resultant increase in plasma testosterone subsequently reduces LH and FSH release.

Actions

As for corticosteroids (see Figure 18–2). Tissue selectivity is achieved by the presence of specific soluble protein receptors found in the cytoplasm of target cells. Testosterone passes from the blood into the cell and combines with specific androgen receptors. Following transfer of the receptor-testosterone complex into the nucleus, testosterone interacts with chromatin to produce the metabolic changes essential for androgenic action. Testosterone, and the other endogenous androgens

- are responsible for the full morphologic and functional development of the male reproductive tract, including the accessory glands and external genitalia;
- determine the distribution and growth of hair on the face, body, and pubes, and the initial recession of the male hairline;
- enlarge the larynx and thicken the vocal cords;
- increase protein anabolism and decrease catabolism; and
- improve the ability of muscles to work, by increasing their number, thickness, and tensile strength.

Pharmacokinetics

Testosterone cannot be given orally, because it is rapidly inactivated during its first pass through the liver. It must be IM injected as the propionate, enanthate, or cypionate esters.

Methyltestosterone can be taken orally or sublingually. Other orally-effective androgens are fluoxymesterone, mesterolone, oxandrolone, and stanozolol.

Uses

Replacement Therapy
Used in patients with **hypogonadism** due to testicular failure.

Given at puberty to males with **hypopituitarism**.

Anemia
Used to **stimulate erythropoiesis** in patients with hypoplastic anemia, the anemia of cancer, red cell aplasia, hemolytic anemias, and anemias related to renal failure, lymphomas, leukemias, and myeloid metaplasias.

Cancer
Used for **recurrent and metastatic carcinoma of the breast**. The response is much better in tumors containing estrogen receptors and/or progesterone receptors.

Anabolic Effects
The androgens ethylestrenol, methylandrostenolone, and stanozolol are used for their anabolic effects to help **postoperative recovery** and to **treat chronic debilitating disease**.

Use in athletes cannot be condoned.

Adverse Effects

Women taking androgens experience **menstrual irregularities**. **Masculinization** can also be seen in females.

- Seen first as acne, growth of facial hair, deepening of voice, and later as the male pattern of baldness.
- Marked development of the skeletal muscle and veins; hypertrophy of the clitoris may subsequently ensue.

Salt and **water retention** because androgens increase renal Na^+, Cl^-, and H_2O reabsorption.

Androgens can cause **biliary stasis**, leading to jaundice and hepatic andenocarcinoma.

Daily use of androgens can decrease FSH and LH in males, resulting in **impotence** and **azoospermia**.

ANTIANDROGENS

Finasteride

Actions

Finasteride is a competitive and specific inhibitor of 5-alpha-reductase, an intracellular enzyme that metabolizes testosterone into the more potent androgen, dihydrotestosterone.

Uses

Finasteride is used to treat symptomatic benign prostatic hyperplasia. It may cause regression of the enlarged prostate and improve blood flow and the symptoms associated with benign prostatic hyperplasia.

Adverse Effects

Finasteride is well tolerated. The most frequent reactions are impotence (3.7%), decreased libido (3.3%), and decreased volume of ejaculate (2.8%).

Antipsychotic Drugs

TYPICAL OR TRADITIONAL ANTIPSYCHOTIC DRUGS (TABLE 20–1)

Actions

Typical antipsychotic drugs block dopamine D_2, histamine H_1, muscarinic, and alpha$_1$-adrenergic receptors (Table 20–1, Figures 20–1 and 20–2).

Table 20–1
Typical and Atypical Antipsychotic Drugs

Typical Antipsychotics	Atypical Antipsychotic
1. *Low-Potency Phenothiazines* 　　Chlorpromazine 　　Mesoridazine 　　Promazine 　　Thioridazine	Clozapine Olanzepine Respiridone
2. *Mid/High-Potency Phenothiazines* 　　Fluphenazine 　　Fluspirilene 　　Perphenazine 　　Prochlorperazine 　　Pimozide 　　Trifluoperazine 3. *Mid/High-Potency Thioxanthene* 　　Thiothixene 4. *Mid/High-Potency Butrophenone* 　　Haloperidol 5. *Mid/High-Potency Dibenzoxazepine* 　　Loxapine	

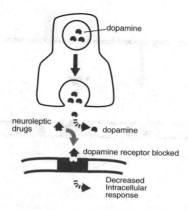

Figure 20–1 Dopamine-blocking actions of antipsychotic drugs. (After Neuroleptic Drugs in: Lippincott's Illustrated Reviews. Eds Harvey RA, Champe PC. New York: Lippincott, 1992.)

Block of Dopamine (D_2)-Receptors in the Brain by Typical Antipsychotics accounts for their:

1. **Antipsychotic actions.** The block of D_2-receptors in the mesolimbic-mesocortical area of the brain is believed to play a major role in controlling the positive symptoms of schizophrenia (eg, irritability, hallucinations, and delusions).

2. **Extrapyramidal effects.** The parkinsonian effects, dystonic reactions, akathisia, and tardive dyskinesia, result from a blockade of D_2-receptors in the nigrostriatal pathway.

3. **Hypersecretion of prolactin.** The hypersecretion of prolactin produced by typical antipsychotics is due to a block of D_2-receptors in the pituitary, which mediate the effects of the prolactin inhibitory factor. Blocking D_2-receptors increases prolactin release, which can result in amenorrhea, infertility, and impotence.

4. **Antiemetic actions.** Stimulation of D_2-receptors in the chemoreceptor area of the medulla oblongata of the brain plays a pivotal role in the nausea and vomiting produced by many drugs and chemicals. The antiemetic action of many typical antipsychotics results from a block of these receptors.

Block of Histamine₁ (H_1)-Receptors (Antihistaminic Effects)

Higher doses of phenothiazines, such as chlorpromazine, are more likely to produce pronounced sedation. This is at least partly due to a block of H_1-receptors.

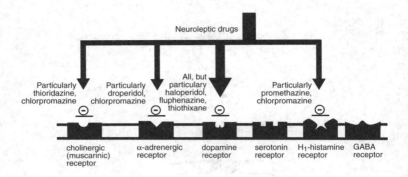

Figure 20–2 Blocking actions of antipsychotic drugs. GABA = gamma-aminobutyric acid. (After Neuroleptic Drugs in: Lippincott's Illustrated Reviews. Eds Harvey RA, Champe PC. New York: Lippincott, 1992.)

Block of Muscarinic Receptors

The ability of typical antipsychotics to block muscarinic receptors in the body (see Chapter 4) explains the dry mouth, constipation, urinary retention, and cycloplegia produced by these drugs.

Block of Alpha₁-Adrenergic Receptors

By blocking α_1-adrenergic receptors, some typical antipsychotics dilate arterioles, decreasing peripheral resistance and blood pressure, and veins, reducing venous return and causing orthostatic hypotension (see Chapter 6).

Uses

Psychoses are the major indications for these drugs. Antipsychotic drug therapy is the most effective treatment for the acute-onset phase in schizophrenia or schizophreniform disorder. These drugs may also be very helpful in the prevention or recurrence of acute schizophrenic disturbances. Typical antipsychotic drugs are less effective in the chronic phase of schizophrenia, particularly with such negative symptoms as anergia, low motivation, and flat affect. These drugs are also used to treat other psychoses, including **mania and paranoia.** Despite differences in potency, all typical antipsychotic drugs are equally effective in equivalent doses. The drug of choice is usually the one the patient can best tolerate (see Adverse Effects below).

Typical antipsychotic drugs are combined with lithium to treat the acute manic episodes of **bipolar affective disorders** and to prevent recurrences.

Organic mental syndromes, usually manifested as either delirium or dementia, can be treated with typical antipsychotic drugs.

Nausea and vomiting resulting from the use of anticancer drugs, radiation, estrogens, tetracyclines, and narcotics, and from uremia, can be treated with typical antipsychotic drugs. Only thioridazine seems devoid of antiemetic effects. Antipsychotics are not effective in controlling motion sickness.

Adverse Effects

CNS depression, which may be due to H_1-receptor antagonism, is common with all typical antipsychotics and pronounced after large doses of the low-potency phenothiazines.

Anticholinergic effects can lead to mydriasis, cycloplegia, dry mouth, retention or difficulty in urination, and constipation. Muscarinic block can also cause a toxic confusional state.

Alpha₁-adrenergic receptor blockade can cause orthostatic hypotension, impotence, and failure to ejaculate. Orthostatic hypotension is more prevalent with the low-potency antipsychotics.

Inhibition of D_2-pituitary receptors increases prolactin release, causing amenorrhea, infertility, and impotence.

Hypersensitivity reactions include obstructive jaundice and blood dyscrasias, manifested as leukopenia, leukocytosis, and eosinophilia.

Skin pigmentation, seen most often with chlorpromazine and other low-potency drugs, is apparently the result of the accumulation of the antipsychotic and its metabolites in the skin. Photosensitivity, most common with long-term chlorpromazine treatment, usually appears in the form of hypersensitivity to the sun and severe sunburn.

Neuroleptic malignant syndrome is a rare, but serious, syndrome of unknown cause. Its symptoms include tachycardia, sweating, rigidity, fevers, fluctuations in blood pressure, seizure, or coma.

Extrapyramidal symptoms (EPS) are of great concern. Dopamine (DA) and acetylcholine (Ach) are physiologic antagonists in the striatum of the brain, with DA acting as an inhibitor and Ach as an excitatory neurotransmitter. Because typical antipsychotics block D_2-receptors, they disturb the normal balance between Ach and DA in the brain. As a result, the excitatory effects of Ach are seen unfettered by the inhibitory actions of DA. The EPS of typical antipsychotics can be divided into the direct and indirect consequences of the D_2 block (Table 20–2).

ATYPICAL ANTIPSYCHOTIC DRUGS

Clozapine, olanzapine, and risperidone are often referred to as "atypical antipsychotics" because their pharmacologic and therapeutic effects differ

Table 20–2
Extrapyramidal Effects of Traditional Antipsychotics

Direct Effects of the Block of DA Receptors	Indirect Effect of the Block of DA Receptors
Parkinsonian effects — involve a decrease or slowing of voluntary movements associated with masked faces, tremor at rest, and a decrease in reciprocal arm movements when walking. Seen in about 13% of patients on typical antipsychotics, parkinsonian effects may appear as early as 5 days or as late as 1 month after treatment begins. Reducing the dose of the antipsychotic or adding an anticholinergic-antiparkinsonian drug (see Chapter 24) decreases the severity of the syndrome	**Tardive dyskinesia** — occurs in 10 to 40% of patients receiving long-term typical antipsychotic drug therapy and is characterized by involuntary and lateral jaw movements and fly-catching movements of the tongue. Choreiform-like movements, characterized by quick, jerky, purposeless movements of the extremities, may also occur. Tardive dyskinesia results indirectly from a block of D_2-receptors. The block of D_2-receptors by these drugs increases both the turnover and stores of DA within nerve terminals. In time, the block of D_2-receptors also results in the formation of new and supersensitive D_2-receptors. Tardive dyskinesia results from the overstimulation of these new D_2-receptors. Because tardive dyskinesia is caused by overstimulation of new supersensitive D_2-receptors and not cholinergic predominance, it does not respond to anticholinergic-antiparkinsonian drugs. Tardive dyskinesia may occur within the first year of treatment or take considerably longer to appear. The risk increases with duration of treatment and the use of high-potency drugs
Dystonic reactions — include facial grimacing, torticollis, oculogyric crisis, difficulty in speech and swallowing, and uncoordinated, spastic movements of the body and limbs. Seen in 12% of patients on typical antipsychotics, these effects usually appear 1 – 5 days after starting treatment. Giving an anticholinergic-antiparkinsonian drug decreases the severity of the syndrome	
Akathisia — is the inability to sit quietly. Seen in 37% of patients treated with typical antipsychotics, it is characterized as restlessness, pacing, and insomnia. An anticholinergic-antiparkinsonian drug should reduce the symptoms	

DA = dopamine.

significantly from those of the typical or traditional antipsychotics. For many patients, the atypical drugs provide relief previously not available with the older drugs and cause less EPS than typical antipsychotics.

1. Clozapine

Actions

Clozapine differs from typical antipsychotics in its ability to block dopamine$_4$- (D_4) receptors. This action presumably explains its antipsychotic effects. Clozapine is a relatively poor D_2-receptor blocker. It has the least affinity of any antipsychotic drug for D_2 receptors in the caudate nucleus, and this probably accounts for the fact that it does not produce EPS.

Uses

Clozapine is effective in controlling both positive symptoms (eg, irritability, hallucinations, and delusions) and negative symptoms (eg, social disinterest or incompetence and poor personal hygiene) of schizophrenia and other psychoses. Compared with other antipsychotics, clozapine appears to be particularly useful in the treatment of severely disturbed, treatment-refractory patients, in whom it has a 40 to 60% success rate. Clozapine may also be effective in other unresponsive psychotic mood or schizoaffective disorders. In addition, because of the very low risk of EPS with this drug, a trial of clozapine is clearly indicated for patients in whom EPS (including tardive dyskinesia) are severe and intolerable with other agents.

Adverse Effects

Agranulocytosis occurs in 1 to 2% of patients, usually in the first 6 months of treatment. Although this reaction also occurs with other antipsychotics, it is more prominent with clozapine. Clients must have a normal white blood cell (WBC) and differential count prior to starting therapy. Subsequently, a WBC and differential count must be carried out weekly throughout treatment and for at least 4 weeks after stopping clozapine.

Other adverse effects include drowsiness or sedation (40%), hypersalivation (30%), tachycardia (25%; persistent in 10%), dizziness (20%), and orthostatic hypotension (9%). Weight gain, transient fever, and seizures can occur with clozapine.

2. Olanzapine

Actions

Olanzapine selectively inhibits mesolimbic dopaminergic pathways. Because olanzapine does not inhibit nigrostriatal dopaminergic activity, its EPS are kept to a minimum. Olanzapine's low incidence of side effects is also due to its greater affinity for serotonin$_{2A}$/5-hydroxytryptamine$_{2A}$ (5-HT$_{2A}$) receptors over D$_2$-receptors.

Uses

Olanzapine appears to control the positive, negative, and affective (mood) symptoms of schizophrenia. Olanzapine also demonstrates fewer EPS than typical antipsychotics.

Adverse Effects

Somnolence appears to be the most frequent adverse effect (about 25% of patients). Other possible adverse effects include dizziness, headache, agitation, and rhinitis.

3. Risperidone

Actions

Risperidone blocks both D$_2$ and 5-HT$_2$–receptors. The balanced antagonism of both types of receptors is the basis for risperidone's superior therapeutic efficacy and reduced potential for inducing EPS.

Risperidone also inhibits α_1-adrenergic receptors and H$_1$-histaminergic receptors. As a result of its inhibition of α_1-receptors, risperidone can produce a dose-related fall in blood pressure and reflex tachycardia.

Risperidone changes sleep architecture by promoting deep slow-wave sleep, thereby improving sleeping patterns. This effect is most likely due to risperidone's blockade of 5-HT–receptors.

Uses

Risperidone is used to manage both the positive and negative symptoms of schizophrenia. Its ability to manage the negative symptoms is most significant and, along with its increased safety, serves to set risperidone apart from the typical antipsychotics.

Adverse Effects

Asthenia, sedation, and difficulty in concentrating are the most common adverse effects. Others include orthostatic hypotension, reflex tachycardia, elevation of prolactin levels, weight gain, and sexual dysfunction. In patients taking recommended doses of risperidone, the incidence of EPS is only slightly higher than placebo.

21

Drugs for Mood Disorders

TREATMENT OF DEPRESSION

1. Tricyclic Antidepressants

Actions

Tricyclic antidepressants (TCAs) and maprotiline, a drug that is pharmacologically similar to TCAs, elevate mood; increase physical activity and the activities of daily living; improve appetite and sleep patterns; and reduce morbid preoccupation in 60 to 70% of patients with major depression (Table 21–1). These effects often begin gradually (1 to 6 weeks). The means by which these drugs increase mood is not clearly understood. The central and peripheral actions of TCAs include

Table 21–1
Sedative and Anticholinergic Effects of Some Tricyclic Antidepressants and Maprotiline

Name	Sedation	Anticholinergic Effects
Imipramine	++	++
Clomipramine	++	++
Desipramine	+	+
Amitriptyline	+++	+++
Nortriptyline	++	++
Doxepin	+++	+++
Protriptyline	0	++
Maprotiline	+++	+/0

0 = none; + = slight; ++ = moderate; +++ = high

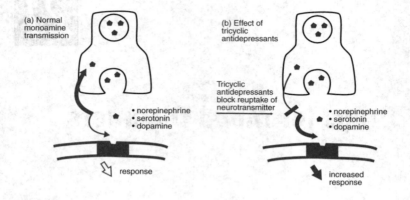

Figure 21–1 Mechanism of action of tricyclic antidepressants. (After Harvey RA, Champe PC. Lippincott's illustrated review: pharmacology. New York: J.P. Lippincott, 1992, p 120.)

A. Block of Neuronal Reuptake of Norepinephrine (NE) and/or 5-Hydroxytryptamine (Serotonin, 5-HT) in the Brain (Figure 21–1).

1. *Inhibition of Reuptake*

The ability of TCAs to inhibit NE and possibly 5-HT reuptake may account for their therapeutic effects. Neuronal reuptake is the major physiologic mechanism for removing NE and 5-HT from their receptors. If a drug blocks neuronal reuptake, it raises the concentration of the neurotransmitter around receptors which increases the effect of the neurotransmitter.

2. *Time Between Block of Reuptake and Relief of Depression*

TCAs quickly inhibit NE and possibly 5-HT neuronal reuptake, but they require 1 to 6 weeks to relieve depression. Obviously, blocking reuptake is only the first step in modifying mood.

3. *Down-Regulation of β-Receptors*

It is speculated that the block in NE neuronal reuptake leads to a down-regulation or subsensitization of β-adrenergic receptors. Down-regulation of β-receptors takes 2 or 3 weeks and correlates with relief of depression.

4. *Summary of Sequence of TCA Effects on Central Nervous System (CNS) NE*

The antidepressant effects of TCAs may, at least partly, be attributed to the following sequence of events:

- Inhibition of NE reuptake
- Increase in synaptic concentrations of NE
- Increase of neuronal NE release during normal rates of firing
- Further increase in synaptic concentrations of NE
- Desensitization of postsynaptic β-receptors

5. *Summary of Sequence of TCA Effects on CNS 5-HT*

Some TCAs also inhibit 5-HT reuptake and this may lead to desensitization of 5-HT–receptors.

B. Block of Alpha$_1$ (α_1), Histamine$_1$ (H$_1$), and Muscarinic Receptors

TCAs block α_1-adrenergic receptors, producing orthostatic hypotension; H$_1$-receptors, causing sedation; and muscarinic receptors, resulting in blurred vision, dry mouth, decreased sweating, constipation, urinary retention, and delayed ejaculation. Table 21–1 summarizes the sedative (antihistaminic) and anticholinergic effects of TCAs.

Uses

TCAs are most effective in patients suffering from more severe depression, particularly with greater vegetative disturbance and melancholia. Usually, the more sedative drugs (amitriptyline and doxepin) are preferred for anxious or agitated depressives, while the less sedative drugs (protriptyline) are better for patients with psychomotor withdrawal.

Adverse Effects

Cardiovascular (CV) effects — orthostatic hypotension is the most common CV effect. Other effects seen with increasing doses are palpitations, tachycardia, cardiac arrhythmias, and ECG abnormalities. Ventricular arrhythmias, including fibrillation, can occur with large doses.

    Anticholinergic effects — see above.

    CNS effects — confusion can occur, especially in patients over age 40, and particularly when used with drugs that also block muscarinic receptors. Sedation is common. TCAs can produce tremors.

    Weight gain can also occur with TCAs.

2. Selective Serotonin Reuptake Inhibitors (SSRIs) (Fluoxetine, Fluvoxamine, Nefazodone, Paroxetine, Sertraline)

Actions

SSRIs selectively inhibit 5-HT neuronal reuptake, with little or no effect on NE reuptake. SSRIs also take 1 to 6 weeks to relieve depression.

Uses

SSRIs are used primarily in moderately and severely depressed out-patients. They may be particularly useful

- in patients with concurrent illness such as hypertension, coronary artery disease, prostatic enlargement, or narrow-angle glaucoma;
- in those who cannot tolerate the adverse effects of TCAs; and
- in the elderly.

Adverse Effects

Headache, tremor, nausea, diarrhea, insomnia, agitation, and nervousness are most frequent.

SSRIs may cause either agitation or sedation.

Because SSRIs do not have the anticholinergic, antihistaminic, or α_1-receptor blocking activities of the TCAs, they are less likely to cause orthostatic hypotension, tachycardia, delayed cardiac conduction, seizures, blurred vision, or dry mouth.

Anorgasmia in both men and women and ejaculatory disturbances appear more common with SSRIs than with TCAs.

SSRIs are much safer in an overdose than TCAs, which can cause lethal cardiac toxicity.

3. Monoamine Oxidase Inhibitors (MAOIs) (Phenelzine, Tranylcypromine, Moclobemide)

Actions

Monoamine oxidase (MAO) refers to a group of enzymes widely distributed throughout the body that oxidatively deaminate and inactivate NE, dopamine (DA) and 5-HT. MAOIs increase brain levels of NE, DA and 5-HT (Figure 21–2). They probably relieve depression by this increase in brain NE and/or 5-HT. Enzyme inhibition appears after a few doses; however, the antidepressant effects of MAOIs take 2 to 4 weeks of treatment.

MAOs exists in the body as two isozymes, MAO-A and MAO-B, each with selective substrate and inhibitor characteristics:

- MAO-A preferentially metabolizes NE and 5-HT in the brain.
- MAO-B metabolizes DA in the brain.
- Inhibition of MAO-A, not MAO-B, is important to the antidepressant actions of MAOIs.
- Phenelzine and tranylcypromine inhibit both MAO-A and MAO-B. Moclobemide inhibits only MAO-A.

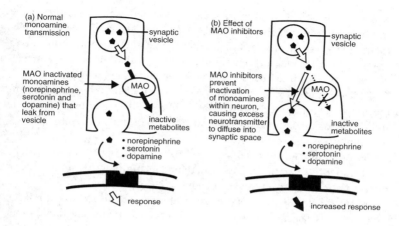

Figure 21–2 Mechanism of action of MAOIs. (After Harvey RA, Champe PC. Lippincott's illustrated review: pharmacology. New York: J.P. Lippincott, 1992, p. 124.)

Uses

MAOIs are usually used only after other antidepressants have failed. Most physicians consider other antidepressants more effective and less toxic than phenelzine and tranylcypromine. Moclobemide appears to be as effective and as well tolerated as TCAs.

Adverse Effects

Phenelzine and tranylcypromine stimulate the CNS to produce tremors, insomnia, and agitation. They also produce orthostatic hypotension, as well as decreasing cholinergic stimulation, resulting in dry mouth, constipation, difficulty in urination, delayed ejaculation, and impotence. A low incidence of hepatotoxicity is also reported with these drugs. Acute overdosage with phenelzine or tranylcypromine is a serious problem. Symptoms include severe fever, agitation, hyperexcitable reflexes, hallucination, and increase or decrease in blood pressure.

Moclobemide is well tolerated. The most common adverse effects are dry mouth, dizziness, headache, somnolence, nausea, and insomnia.

Interaction of MAOIs with Food and Drugs

Tyramine is found in such foods as cheese, beer, wine, pickled herring, snails, chicken liver, and coffee. It is normally metabolized rapidly by MAO-A in the cells of the intestinal wall and liver, and by MAO-B in the liver. Phenelzine and tranylcypromine inhibit both MAO-A and MAO-B, increasing the circulating levels of tyramine, which enters sympathetic nerve endings and releases NE. The resulting generalized vasoconstriction produces a hypertensive crisis. Death can occur from an intracranial hemorrhage.

Moclobemide is safer because tyramine can effectively compete with moclobemide for intestinal and hepatic MAO-A. Moreover, liver MAO-B is still available to inactivate any tyramine that is not metabolized by MAO-A in the intestine or liver.

TCAs should not be used with MAOIs. By reducing both the reuptake of NE and its enzymatic inactivation, their concomitant use can produce a hyperpyretic crisis or severe convulsions.

MAOIs decrease the metabolism and increase the actions of a large number of drugs, such as narcotics, barbiturates, many anesthetics, and anticholinergics.

4. Miscellaneous Antidepressants

A. Trazodone

Actions

Like SSRIs, trazadone inhibits the neuronal reuptake of 5-HT. Trazadone also stimulates the neuronal release of NE, and because of this action chronic trazadone treatment leads to down-regulation (subsensitivity) of β-adrenergic receptors. This action may play a role in the antidepressant effects of trazodone.

Trazadone is relatively free of antimuscarinic and CV adverse effects.

Uses

Trazadone is as effective as amitriptyline in both major and other subsets of depressive disorders. Because of its sedative effect, trazadone is generally more useful in depressive disorders associated with insomnia and anxiety.

Adverse Effects

Trazadone is generally well tolerated. Drowsiness is most common, and mild nausea and vomiting occur less frequently. Trazadone can cause orthostatic hypotension for 4 to 6 hours after ingestion. This can be reduced by giving the drug with food.

B. Venlafaxine

Actions

Venlafaxine is similar to TCAs because it inhibits NE and 5-HT uptake and weakly inhibits DA uptake. In contrast to TCAs, venlafaxine has no affinity for cholinergic, H_1-, or α_1-receptors.

Uses

Venlafaxine is an effective antidepressant.

Adverse Events

Venlafaxine's adverse effects resemble those of SSRIs. Nausea, headache, anxiety, anorexia, nervousness, sweating, dizziness, insomnia, and somnolence are the most common.

C. Bupropion

Actions

Bupropion's mechanism of action is not known. Although it blocks the reuptake of dopamine, this effect is seen only at higher doses than those needed to relieve depression. Bupropion is a weak blocker of 5-HT and NE reuptake, and it does not inhibit MAO.

Uses

Bupropion is used for the treatment of major depression. It appears to be effective without causing the sedation, orthostatic hypotension, weight gain, or sexual dysfunction associated with other antidepressants.

Bupropion is also used as a smoking cessation treatment in conjunction with behavioral modification.

Adverse Effects

Bupropion is generally well tolerated and causes fewer anticholinergic, sedative, or adverse sexual effects than TCAs. It does not cause weight gain and does not affect cardiac conduction or produce orthostatic hypotension. Agitation has been the most frequent reason for stopping the drug. Dry mouth, headache, dizziness, insomnia, anorexia, weight loss, nausea, and constipation have occurred.

The main concern in using bupropion is the risk for seizures. These occur more frequently at higher doses. Caution is used in patients with a history of seizures or cranial trauma, during concurrent use with other medications that may lower the seizure threshold, or when changes in treatment regimens occur.

TREATMENT OF MANIC-DEPRESSIVE ILLNESS (BIPOLAR DISORDER)

Lithium

Actions

Lithium's mechanism of action is not known. Lithium is a positively charged ion, similar to sodium and potassium. It is unclear whether its therapeutic effects have any relationship to the actions of sodium or potassium.

Therapeutic concentrations of lithium have no noticeable effects in normal individuals. Lithium differs from other psychotropic drugs in that it is not a sedative, euphoriant, or depressant. It corrects sleep patterns in manic patients but has no primary action on sleep itself, other than perhaps a small decrease in rapid eye movement (REM) sleep.

Lithium carbonate is well absorbed from the intestine, producing sharp peaks in serum concentrations. The use of a sustained-release lithium carbonate preparation can reduce the frequency of absorption-related side effects.

Lithium is excreted by the kidney, with a half-life of 17 to 36 hours. Lithium elimination is reduced in patients with renal impairment. Reducing sodium intake increases the renal reabsorption of lithium; therefore, patients on lithium should not be given a low sodium diet.

Uses

Lithium carbonate is used to treat mania. Lithium requires 1 to 3 weeks of treatment before it is effective. When mania is mild, lithium alone may suffice. In more severe cases, an antipsychotic drug, usually haloperidol or chlorpromazine, is also given (see Chapter 20). After adequate serum levels of lithium have been reached, the antipsychotic may be carefully withdrawn. During the depressive phase, lithium may be combined with a TCA or bupropion.

Prophylactic lithium treatment is considered the therapy of choice to prevent recurrences of manic-depressive disorder.

Lithium is contraindicated in patients with significant CV or renal disease. It is also contraindicated in severely debilitated or dehydrated patients, and in patients with sodium depletion, brain damage, or those requiring low sodium intake.

Adverse Effects

Lithium has a low therapeutic index and reaches toxic levels quickly. Lithium serum levels should be measured frequently during stabilization and routinely during maintenance. For many patients, serum concentrations of 0.6 to 0.7 mmol/L are effective and well tolerated. Mild to moderate toxic effects occur at 1.5 to 2.0 mmol/L and moderate to severe reactions above 2.0 mmol/L.

Nausea, lethargy, and fatigue may occur in the first weeks of treatment, even when serum concentrations are in the recommended range. Fine tremor of the hand is common, especially during initial treatment. As the concentration of lithium increases, the fine tremor may become coarse and ataxia, dysarthria, loss of coordination, difficulty in concentration, and mild disorientation may be established. Other signs of neurologic toxicity include muscle twitching and fasciculations in the limbs, hands, and face, together with nystagmus, dizziness, and visual disturbances. The signs of severe toxicity are restlessness, confusion, nystagmus, epileptic convulsion, delirium, and eventually, coma and death.

Polyuria and polydipsia occur in 15 to 40% of patients. These do not bother most patients. Toxic renal effects, including tubular lesions, interstitial fibrosis, and decreased creatinine clearance are uncommon but have been reported following chronic lithium treatment. Lithium can also produce nephrogenic diabetes insipidus.

Lithium can cause euthyroid goitre, hypothyroidism, with or without goitre, and abnormal endocrine test results.

22

Anxiolytics and Hypnotics

BENZODIAZEPINES

Actions

Benzodiazepines reduce anxiety by depressing the limbic system. The limbic system, composed of the septal region of the brain, the amygdala, the hippocampus, and the hypothalamus, is important in determining an individual's emotional and autonomic response to situations.

Benzodiazepines depress the limbic system by facilitating the action of γ-aminobutyric acid (GABA). Binding of GABA to its receptors inhibits the formation of action potentials and depresses neuronal function. Benzodiazepines bind to specific, high-affinity sites on the cell membrane, which are separate from, but adjacent to, the receptors for GABA. This binding of benzodiazepines to their receptors enhances the affinity of GABA receptors for GABA. This results in greater depression of neuronal function.

Pharmacokinetics

Benzodiazepines are usually absorbed quickly and then metabolized. The metabolic inter-relationship of the benzodiazepines is complex (Figure 22–1 and Table 22–1). Their half-lives range from 2 to 3 hours for triazolam to approximately 50 to 100 hours for diazepam and flurazepam. Chlordiazepoxide, ketazolam, and diazepam are active themselves and are also metabolized to active compounds. The half-lives given for these drugs take into account the duration of action of the metabolites, as well as the parent compounds.

Because benzodiazepines are often prescribed for prolonged periods of time, their long-term pharmacokinetics are important. When a drug is taken chronically, it requires about 5 half-lives to reach steady state. Therefore, drugs with long half-lives, such as diazepam, require 2 to 3 weeks before they

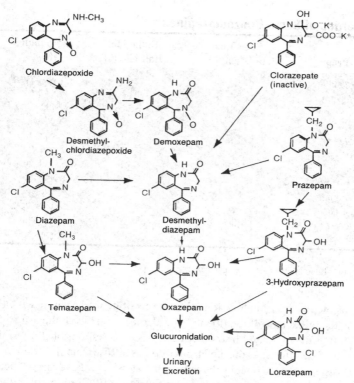

Figure 22–1 Benzodiazepine metabolism. (After Morgan JP. Alcohol and drug abuse. Curriculum guide for pharmacology faculty. Rockville, MD: U.S. Department of Health and Human Services, 1985:44.)

reach plateau levels, and patients may not experience their full effects until treatment has continued for this length of time. Other benzodiazepines with shorter half-lives, such as oxazepam, reach plateau concentrations within 1 to 3 days and maximum effects are seen sooner.

Once treatment with a drug is stopped, it is eliminated from the body in relation to its half-life. Thus, the effects of diazepam last long after the drug is stopped. The actions of lorazepam, with a half-life of 12 to 15 hours, disappear faster. The rapid elimination of a benzodiazepine from the body following prolonged treatment can be a mixed blessing. Although the patient may not be bothered with the "hangover" effects of the drug, rapid elimination of the benzodiazepine often causes rebound excitation and a request for another prescription. Patients on shorter-acting benzodiazepines may be more likely to become dependent on these drugs.

Although metabolic inactivation is important in determining the duration of action of a benzodiazepine during long-term treatment, it is not

Table 22–1
Properties of Some Benzodiazepines

Drug	Peak Time of Effect (h)	Biological Half-Life (h)	Therapeutic Use*
Triazolam	2	2-3	Hypnotic
Oxazepam	1-4	4-13	Anxiolytic
Temazepam	0.8-1.4	8-10	Hypnotic
Bromazepam	1-4	12	Anxiolytic
Alprazolam	1-2	6-20	Anxiolytic
Lorazepam	1-6	12-15	Anxiolytic
Chlordiazepoxide	2-4	20-24†	Anxiolytic
Nitrazepam	2	26	Hypnotic
Clorazepate	1-2	48†	Anxiolytic
Ketazolam	?	50†	Anxiolytic
Diazepam	1.5-2	50-100†	Anxiolytic
Flurazepam	1	50-100†	Hypnotic

*Refers to anxiolytic and hypnotic uses only.
†Refers to half-life of drug plus active metabolites.

responsible for deciding how long the actions of benzodiazepine will last during the initial days of treatment. Instead, the rate at which the drug diffuses out of the brain and into other body tissues is responsible for terminating its CNS effects. As most benzodiazepines diffuse from the brain into other tissues at approximately the same rate following initial doses, all benzodiazepines should have approximately the same initial duration of action. For example:

- Triazolam is rapidly inactivated by metabolism and has a half-life of 2 to 3 hours.
- Flurazepam is metabolized very rapidly to its active metabolite, N-desalkylflurazepam, which is slowly inactivated and has a half-life of 50 to 100 hours.
- Despite these differences, both drugs have approximately the same initial duration of action because triazolam and N-desalkylflurazepam diffuse out of the brain at about the same rate during the initial nights of treatment.

If flurazepam is given for several nights, N-desalkylflurazepam levels increase in blood and other tissues because it is slowly metabolized. With higher blood levels, less N-desalkylflurazepam is less able to diffuse out of the brain and its hypnotic effects last longer.

Because triazolam is rapidly metabolized, chronic treatment should not lead to accumulation. As a result, triazolam should have a shorter duration of action than flurazepam, when both drugs are given night after night.

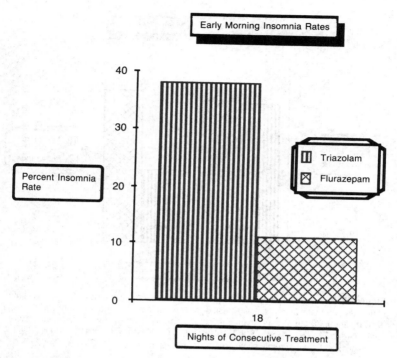

Figure 22–2 Early morning insomnia with triazolam and flurazepam. Patients were treated nightly with 0.5 mg of triazolam or 30 mg of flurazepam. Early morning insomnia rate was measured during nights 16 to 18. (After Kales A, Soldatos CR, Bixler EO, Kales JC. Early morning insomnia with rapidly eliminated benzodiazepines. Science 1983; 220:95–97.)

The short half-life of triazolam means that patients on chronic triazolam may experience early morning insomnia (Figure 22–2). However, they should not have significant daytime sedation. In contrast, patients on chronic flurazepam experience daytime "hangover," because significant amounts of N-desalkylflurazepam remain in the brain during the waking hours.

Tolerance and Dependence

Tolerance develops to benzodiazepines. Figure 22–3 shows that patients spent more time awake after 18 nights of treatment with triazolam than they did after 7 nights. The percentage change in mean wake time for flurazepam did not change between week 1 and week 3 because the long half-life of N-desalkylflurazepam resulted in its accumulation in the brain, minimizing the consequences of tissue tolerance.

Dependence to benzodiazepines is also common. Figure 22–4 demonstrates

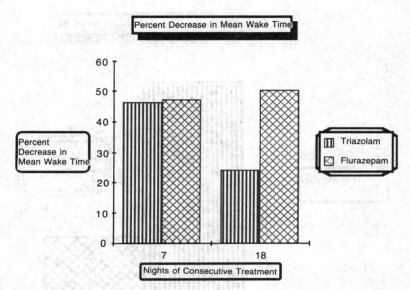

Figure 22–3 Change in percent mean wake time from control values during the first 6 hours of night for triazolam- and flurazepam-treated patients. Patients were treated nightly with 0.5 mg of triazolam or 30 mg of flurazepam. Percentage change in mean wake time was measured during nights 5 to 7 and nights 16 to 18. (After Kales A, Soldatos CR, Bixler EO, Kales JC. Early morning insomnia with rapidly eliminated benzodiazepines. Science 1983; 220:95–97.)

- the development of tolerance to triazolam between days 5 to 7 and 16 to 18, and
- the appearance of rebound insomnia when patients stopped taking the hypnotic.

Drugs with shorter half-lives are more likely to leave the patient with rebound insomnia. This may lead to dependence on the drug and demands for repeat prescription. The danger of drug dependence is greater with hypnotics having shorter half-lives.

Uses

Anxiety disorders, including panic and generalized anxiety, are the main uses for benzodiazepines. These drugs may also be used for brief periods in stress-related conditions, but this must be done with some caution. A "benzodiazepine crutch" to allay anxiety should be employed for shorter periods only.

Insomnia is the second major use for benzodiazepines. Ideally, a hypnotic should produce sleep quickly, work throughout the night, and have no hangover effects. Although all hypnotics work quickly, short-acting

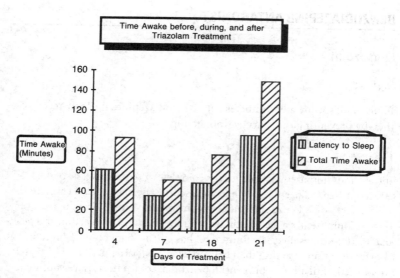

Figure 22–4 Effect of triazolam on the induction and maintenance of sleep. Patients received 4 nights of placebo therapy prior to triazolam on day 4. Baseline data on Days 2 to 4. Day 5 was the first day of triazolam. Day 7 – effects of triazolam on latency to sleep and total time awake during days 5 to 7. Day 18 – effect of triazolam on latency to sleep and total time awake during days 16 to 18. Triazolam treatment was stopped after day 18. Day 21 — effect of withdrawal from triazolam on day 19 to 21. (After Kales A, Sharf MB, Kales JD. Rebound insomnia: a new clinical syndrome. Science 1978; 201:1039–1041.)

benzodiazepines are frequently not effective during the entire night, and long-acting drugs leave patients with a morning hangover. Furthermore, tolerance to these drugs develops rapidly, particularly when a short-acting drug is used. Finally, many patients experience rebound insomnia when short-acting benzodiazepines are stopped.

Adverse Effects

CNS depression (fatigue, drowsiness, and feelings of detachment) is the major benzodiazepine adverse effect. Elderly patients are particularly prone to headache, dizziness, ataxia, confusion, and disorientation. Psychological impairment can occur. Physiologic dependence (characterized by anxiety, agitation, restlessness, insomnia, and tension) following drug withdrawal can also be seen. Although overdosage is common, few patients die. Unless consumed with another CNS depressant or a narcotic, benzodiazepines rarely kill.

BENZODIAZEPINE ANTAGONIST

Flumazenil

Actions

Flumazenil specifically competes with benzodiazepines for their receptors, thereby preventing these drugs from acting.

Uses

Intravenous flumazenil is used for the complete or partial reversal of the CNS effects of benzodiazepines. It may be used in anesthesia, to terminate the CNS effects of a benzodiazepine, and in intensive care, to manage overdosage. Flumazenil's effects begin within 1 to 2 minutes of injection and peak in 6 to 10 minutes. Because flumazenil has a half-life of about 1 hour and a shorter duration of action than benzodiazepines, patients should be closely monitored until all possible central benzodiazepine effects have subsided.

Adverse Effects

Flumazenil can cause nausea, dizziness, headache, blurred vision, increased sweating and anxiety, and may provoke a panic attack in some patients. The drug can cause convulsions in patients who are physically dependent on benzodiazepines or who are taking them to control epilepsy.

NONBENZODIAZEPINE ANXIOLYTICS AND HYPNOTICS

1. Buspirone

Actions

Buspirone's mechanism of action is not clear. Although buspirone shares some of the antianxiety properties of benzodiazepines, it is not an anticonvulsant or muscle relaxant and it does not bind to the benzodiazepine GABA receptor.

Uses

Buspirone is used for the short-term symptomatic relief of excessive anxiety in patients with generalized anxiety disorder.

Adverse Effects

The most common adverse reactions are dizziness, headache, drowsiness, and nausea.

2. Zopiclone

Actions

Zopiclone is a short-acting hypnotic. Zopiclone is rapidly absorbed and extensively metabolized with a half-life of 5 hours.

Uses

Zopiclone is useful for the short-term management of insomnia characterized by difficulty in falling asleep and/or early morning awakenings. Zopiclone reduces sleep latency and increases sleep duration. It produces minimal morning residual effects and does not reduce daytime performance. Zopiclone causes either no, or only slight, psychomotor impairment. Tolerance to zopiclone does not develop over eight weeks of therapy. Rebound insomnia is not marked when patients stop zopiclone. Zopiclone does not significantly affect sleep architecture. There is no evidence that zopiclone produces drug dependence.

Adverse Effects

The adverse effects of zopiclone differ qualitatively from those of the various benzodiazepines. Bitter taste is the most common adverse reaction to zopiclone. Severe drowsiness and/or impaired coordination are signs of drug intolerance or excessive doses.

3. Barbiturates (Amobarbital, Butabarbital, Pentobarbital, Secobarbital)

Actions

Barbiturates potentiate GABA-mediated inhibitory process in the CNS to produce muscle relaxant, anticonvulsant, sedative, and hypnotic effects. Barbiturates alter psychological functions, particularly complex tasks, and especially fine points of judgement. Increasing doses lead to progressive impairment of brain function, culminating with respiratory failure.

Uses

The availability of safer drugs (see above) has eliminated any need for the continued use of barbiturates as anxiolytics (sedatives) or hypnotics.

Adverse Effects

CNS depression is the major adverse effect. Patients may experience drowsiness, confusion, or even psychosis. Other signs of CNS depression include nystagmus, dysarthria, and motor incoordination. The elderly are particularly at risk for ataxia and confusion. Paradoxic excitation may also occur. Overdosage can cause respiratory failure.

4. Chloral Hydrate

Actions

Chloral hydrate works quickly and has a relatively short duration of action.

Uses

Chloral hydrate is frequently used as a hypnotic in pediatrics and geriatrics. It is better suited for putting people to sleep than it is for keeping them asleep.

Adverse Effects

Chloral hydrate produces gastric irritation. Because the drug depresses the CNS, it produces all the effects consistent with depression of the brain. If large doses are taken, death can occur as a result of respiratory failure.

Part 7 Drugs for the Treatment of Neurologic Disorders

23

Drugs for the Treatment of Epilepsy

Epilepsy is a symptom of excessive temporary neuronal discharge due to intracranial or extracranial causes. It is characterized clinically by discrete episodes, which tend to be recurrent, in which there is a disturbance of movement, sensation, behavior, perception and/or consciousness (Sutherland and Eadie).*

ETIOLOGIC AND SEIZURE PATTERN CLASSIFICATIONS OF EPILEPSY (TABLES 23–1 AND 23–2)

Table 23–1
Etiologic Classification of Epilepsy

Primary Epilepsy	Secondary Epilepsy
The cause is not known; thus it is also called idiopathic epilepsy Characterized by major (grand mal) or minor seizures (petit mal, myoclonic, and akinetic seizures)	Also called symptomatic epilepsy, secondary epilepsy can result from either intracranial causes, such as cerebral tumours, cerebrovascular occlusive disease, or head injury; or extracranial problems, such anoxia, uremia, or eclampsia

*After Sutherland JM and Eadie MJ. The epilepsies: modern diagnosis and treatment. 3rd ed. New York: Churchill Livingstone, 1980.

193

Table 23–2
Seizure Pattern Classification of Epilepsy

Generalized Seizures	Partial Seizures	Unclassified Seizures
Bilateral symmetrical seizures without local onset, clinically: (a) Absence seizures (petit mal) (b) Bilateral myoclonus (c) Infantile spasms (d) Clonic seizures (e) Tonic seizures (f) Tonic-clonic seizures (grand mal) (g) Akinetic seizures	Seizures beginning locally with: (a) Elementary symptomatology, • Motor • Sensory • Autonomic • Compound forms (b) Complex symptomatology, • Impaired consciousness • Complex hallucinations • Affective symptoms • Automatism (repetitive, purposeless behaviours) (c) Partial seizures becoming generalized tonic-clonic seizures.	Seizures that cannot be classified because of incomplete data

Classification suggested by the International League Against Epilepsy. (After Sutherland JM, Eadie MJ. The epilepsies: modern diagnosis and treatment. 3rd ed. New York: Churchill Livingstone, 1980.)

Symptoms of Epilepsy (Figure 23–1)

The symptoms of epilepsy depend on
1. the site of the epileptic focus, and
2. the degree to which it spreads.

Most antiepileptic drugs reduce the spread of the abnormal electrical impulse.

CHOICE OF DRUG THERAPY

Choice of drug therapy is determined by the kinds of seizures experienced (Table 23–3).

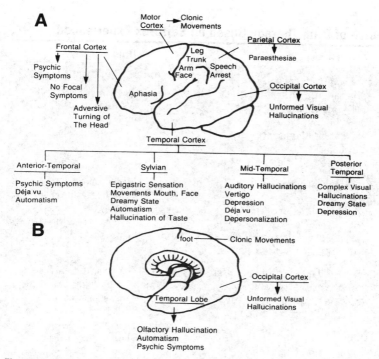

Figure 23–1 Manifestations of partial (symptomatic, cortical) epilepsy. (After Sutherland JM, Eadie MJ). The Epilepsies: Modern Diagnosis and Treatment. 3rd ed. New York: Churchill Livingstone, 1980:27.)

DRUGS EFFECTIVE AGAINST GENERALIZED TONIC-CLONIC SEIZURES

1. Phenytoin

Actions and Pharmacokinetics

Phenytoin appears to prevent the spread of seizure activity in the cerebrum by reducing sodium transport across cell membranes. Phenytoin is slowly absorbed from the GI tract. Elimination depends on hepatic metabolism. At low doses, the drug has a half-life of 24 hours. As the dosage increases, the metabolic pathways for its inactivation become progressively more saturated, and the half-life of phenytoin increases. Relatively small increases in dose can produce significant increases in plasma concentrations and drug-related toxicity. Measuring phenytoin plasma levels is valuable in adjusting the dose. Plasma concentrations of phenytoin between 10 and 20 µg/mL (39.6 – 79.2 µmol/L) are often effective without causing undue toxicity.

Table 23–3

Choice of Drug Therapy Based on Seizures Experienced

Type of Seizure	Drug Therapy
Petit mal (absence) seizures are relatively uncommon and begin in childhood. Patients experience recurrent, brief, sudden interruptions of consciousness without falling and have minimal twitching around the face and eyes	Drugs of first choice are valproic acid, sodium valproate, divalproex sodium, or ethosuximide. Clonazepam is an alternative drug
Myoclonic seizures are characterized by bilateral myoclonic jerks of the limbs, face and trunk that, if severe, may throw the patient to the ground. There may be brief lapses of consciousness	Corticosteroids or corticotrophin may stop these seizures and prevent mental deterioration. If they fail, clonazepam, valproic acid, or nitrazepam may control the seizures, but are less likely to prevent mental deterioration
Generalized tonic-clonic seizures may be a manifestation of primary generalized epilepsy or may occur secondary to focal or myoclonic seizures	Carbamazepine or phenytoin are first-line drugs, with phenobarbital, primidone, valproic acid, or sodium valproate serving as second-line drugs Gabapentin, lamotrigine, and vigabatrin are newer adjuvant drugs. Phenobarbital is usually used for the prevention of febrile seizures in infants
Partial or focal epilepsy may activate the deep central grey matter to produce a secondary generalized tonic-clonic seizure	Phenytoin and carbamazepine are first-line drugs. Phenobarbital and primidone are second-line agents. Gabapentin, lamotrigine, and vigabatrin are newer adjuvant drugs
Status epilepticus exists when seizures recur with increasing frequency such that baseline consciousness is not regained between seizures. The patient is considered to be in status epilepticus when seizures last at least 30 minutes. Status epilepticus is a medical emergency	Status epilepticus is usually treated with IV diazepam. Alternatively, lorazepam, phenobarbital, or phenytoin can be administered by IV

IV = intravenous.

Uses

Phenytoin is used orally in adults to control generalized tonic-clonic and psychomotor (grand mal and temporal lobe) seizures and to prevent and treat seizures occurring during or following neurosurgery.

Pediatric formulations are used for the control of generalized tonic-clonic (grand mal) and complex partial (psychomotor and temporal lobe) seizures.

Parenteral phenytoin is used in the treatment of status epilepticus of the grand mal type and the treatment of seizures occurring during or following neurosurgery.

Adverse Effects

Phenytoin can produce gastric irritation, nystagmus, ataxia, diplopia, drowsiness, gum hypertrophy, hirsutism, immunologic abnormalities, skin rashes, hyperglycemia, osteomalacia, lymphadenopathy, leukopenia, megaloblastic anemia, and teratogenicity.

2. Carbamazepine

Actions and Pharmacokinetics

Carbamazepine reduces the propagation of aberrant impulses in the brain. It is absorbed slowly from the GI tract. Its half-life during chronic therapy may range from 8 to over 24 hours. The drug's usual therapy range is 5 to 12 μg/mL (21.1–50.8 μmol/L); however, 15 to 17 μg/mL (63.3–71.7 μmol/L) may be necessary in some patients.

Uses

Carbmazepine's spectrum of activity is similar to phenytoin's. It is a first-line drug for the treatment of generalized tonic-clonic seizures and partial seizures with complex symptomatolgy.

Adverse Effects

Carbamazepine has a low incidence of adverse effects at normal dosages. Most common adverse effects include gastric irritation, diplopia, and blurred vision.

3. Phenobarbital

Actions and Pharmacokinetics

Phenobarbital is a CNS depressant that may act as an antiepileptic by reducing sodium and potassium flux across cell membranes. Phenobarbital is a long-acting barbiturate with a half-life ranging from 60 to 120 hours in adults. The plasma levels that are consistent with good effect and minimal toxicity fall between 15 to 25 μg/mL (64.6–107.7 μmol/L).

Uses

Phenobarbital remains popular for the treatment of tonic-clonic epilepsy, focal seizures, and complex partial seizures. Phenobarbital is also used prophylactically in young children when febrile seizures are feared.

Adverse Effects

CNS depression is the major adverse effect of phenobarbital. Fortunately tolerance to the CNS-depressive effects of phenobarbital occurs when the drug is given chronically. Allergic rashes are reported in 1 to 2% of patients. Prolonged therapy may be associated with folate deficiency, hypocalcemia, and osteomalacia. Hypoprothrombinemia with hemorrhage has been reported in babies delivered from mothers given phenobarbital. This can be treated with vitamin K injections.

4. Primidone

Actions and Pharmacokinetics

Primidone is structurally similar to phenobarbital and has a similar spectrum of antiepileptic activity. Primidone is quickly absorbed and metabolized to phenobarbital and phenylethylmalonamide, both having antiepileptic activity. Because the half-life of primidone is 8 hours and the half-lives of phenobarbital and phenylethylmalonamide are 60 to 120 hours and 24 to 48 hours, respectively, these metabolites accumulate in patients treated with primidone. Effective plasma levels of primidone usually fall between 5 to 10 µg/mL (22.9–45.8 µmol/L). However, phenobarbital plasma levels frequently can be used to guide dosage.

Uses

Primidone is useful in the prevention of grand mal and psychomotor seizures. It may be used alone or in combination with other antiepileptics.

Adverse Effects

Primidone depresses the CNS and can cause sedation, vertigo, nystagmus, ataxia, and diplopia. It can also cause nausea and vomiting. Although serious adverse effects are not common, leukopenia, thrombocytopenia, systemic lupus erythematosus, and lymphadenopathy have been reported. Similar to phenobarbital, primidone may cause maculopapular and morbilliform rashes, hemorrhage in the newborn, megaloblastic anemia, and osteomalacia.

NEWER ADJUVANT DRUGS FOR THE TREATMENT OF GENERALIZED TONIC-CLONIC SEIZURES

1. Gabapentin

Actions and Pharmacokinetics

Gabapentin's mechanism of action is not known. Gabapentin is rapidly absorbed after oral administration, with or without food, achieving maximum plasma concentrations in 2 to 3 hours. Gabapentin is not metabolized and is almost completely excreted by the kidneys, with a half-life of 5 to 7 hours.

Uses

Gabapentin is used as an adjunct therapy for the management of patients who are not satisfactorily controlled by conventional antiepileptic drugs.

Adverse Effects

Gabapentin appears to be well tolerated. Frequently transient mild to moderate somnolence, dizziness, ataxia, fatigue, and nystagmus have been the most common adverse effects.

2. Lamotrigine

Actions and Pharmacokinetics

Lamotrigine may act by stabilizing neuronal voltage-dependent sodium channels, thus reducing the presynaptic release of excitatory amino acids, principally glutamate and aspartate, that are thought to play a role in the generation and spread of epileptic seizures.

Lamotrigine is almost completely absorbed from the GI tract, either with or without food. Plasma concentrations reach a peak in 1.5 to 5 hours. The plasma half-life of a single dose is about 24 hours.

Uses

Lamotrigine is used as an adjunct therapy for the management of adult patients who are not satisfactorily controlled by conventional therapy. It may also be used as monotherapy in adults following withdrawal of concomitant antiepileptic drugs.

Adverse Effects

Dizziness, diplopia, ataxia, blurred vision, nausea, vomiting, and rash have been the common adverse effects when lamotrigine is added to other antiepileptic drugs. Rash has occurred in about 10% of patients and caused about 4% to stop taking the drug. Rarely, serious skin rashes, including Stevens-Johnson syndrome and toxic epidermal necrolysis, have been reported. Although the majority recover following drug withdrawal, some patients experience irreversible scarring, and there have been rare cases of associated death.

3. Vigabatrin

Actions and Pharmacokinetics

The antiepileptic action of vigabatrin has been attributed to its ability to reversibly inhibit γ-aminobutyric acid transferase (GABA-T), the enzyme responsible for the catabolism of the inhibitory neurotransmitter γ-aminobutyric acid (GABA). The resulting increase in GABA is felt to account for vigabatrin's antiepileptic effects.

Vigabatrin is rapidly and almost completely absorbed from the GI tract. Peak plasma concentrations occur within 1 to 2 hours. Vigabatrin is eliminated primarily by renal excretion, with renal clearance of unchanged drug accounting for about 60 to 70% of total clearance.

Uses

Vigabatrin is used for adjunctive management of epilepsy that is not satisfactorily controlled by conventional therapy.

Adverse Effects

Vigabatrin is generally well tolerated. Fatigue, headache, drowsiness, dizziness, depression, weight increase, agitation, tremor, abnormal vision, and amnesia are the most frequent adverse effects.

DRUGS EFFECTIVE AGAINST ABSENCE SEIZURES

1. Ethosuximide

Pharmacokinetics and Uses

Ethosuximide is a first-line drug for the treatment of petit mal epilepsy. With a half-life of 30 hours in children, ethosuximide requires 5 to 7 days of regular treatment to reach steady state. Therapeutic effects are usually obtained with serum levels of 50 to 100 µg/mL (354.2–708.3 µmol/L).

Adverse Effects

Gastric irritation is the most common adverse reaction. Other effects include CNS depression and rashes. Eosinophilia is seen in about 10% of patients. Pancytopenia and aplastic anemia have also occurred. Systemic lupus erythematosus and Stevens-Johnson syndrome have been rarely noted.

2. Valproic Acid, Sodium Valproate, Divalproex Sodium

Pharmacokinetics and Uses

Valproic acid, or sodium valproate, is used alone or adjunctively to treat simple or complex absence seizures, including petit mal. It is also useful in primary tonic-clonic generalized seizures. These drugs may also be used adjunctively in patients with multiple seizure types, which include either absence or tonic-clonic seizures.

Valproic acid and sodium valproate are rapidly absorbed from the GI tract. With a half-life of 6 to 16 hours, they should be administered 3 or 4 times daily. The therapeutic plasma window is 50 to 100 µg/mL (347–694 µmol/L).

Divalproex sodium is a derivative of valproic acid. Provided in enteric-coated tablets, it dissociates into valproic acid in the intestinal tract. The drug may produce less gastric distress than valproic acid.

Adverse Effects

Anorexia, nausea, and vomiting are major deterrents to the use of valproic acid. Taking the drug with food may help.

Minor elevations of serum glutamic oxaloacetic transaminase (SGOT) and serum glutamic pyruvic transaminase (SGPT) and lactate dehydrogenase (LDH) are frequent. Occasionally, laboratory tests also show increases in serum bilirubin and abnormal changes in other liver function tests. These results may reflect serious hepatotoxicity. Hepatic failure resulting in fatalities has occurred. Because children 2 years of age or younger have nearly a 20-fold increase in risk of fatal hepatotoxicity, valproic acid should be used in this age group with extreme caution and as the sole agent. Liver function tests should be performed on patients receiving valproic acid prior to therapy and at frequent intervals thereafter. Care should be observed when administering valproic acid to patients with a prior history of hepatic disease.

Valproic acid may increase the incidence of congenital malformations by 2- to 3-fold in the general population. The increase is largely associated with specific defects (eg, congenital malformations of the heart, cleft lip and/or palate, and neural tube defects).

3. Clonazepam

Uses

Clonazepam is a benzodiazepine (see Chapter 22) that is used alone or as an adjunct in the management of myoclonic and akinetic seizures and petit mal variants.

Adverse Effects

Sedation and drowsiness are the main complaints. Ataxia may also be seen. Alterations in behavior include aggressiveness, argumentativeness, hyperactivity, agitation, depression, euphoria, irritability, forgetfulness, and confusion.

MISCELLANEOUS ANTIEPILEPTICS

1. Clobazam

Uses

Clobazam is a benzodiazepine (see Chapter 22) that has been added to current antiepileptic therapy in patients with refractory seizures. It appears to be a useful adjuvant medication in a variety of seizure types in adults and children.

Adverse Effects

Sedation, drowsiness, fatigue, and dizziness are most common. Ataxia, insomnia, depression, behavioral changes and weight gain have also been reported. Physical and psychological dependence have occurred.

2. Diazepam (See Chapter 22)

Uses

Intravenous diazepam is the recommended treatment for status epilepticus. Repeated injections are required to maintain the high brain levels necessary to terminate status epilepticus.

3. Lorazepam (See Chapter 22)

Uses

Lorazepam is a benzodiazepine. Given by IV, it is effective for the initial treatment of status epilepticus. In this case, the patient must be observed for signs of cardiorespiratory depression, especially when this drug is given with other antiepileptics.

Antiparkinsonian Drugs

CHARACTERISTICS OF PARKINSONISM

Parkinsonism refers to two main disorders with similar clinical symptoms:

1. **Paralysis agitans or idiopathic Parkinson's disease**, which accounts for 90% of the cases, and
2. **Secondary, or symptomatic parkinsonism**, caused by previous infection with the virus of lethargic encephalitis.

Most Prominent Clinical Symptoms

Akinesia is difficulty in initiating movements or modifying ongoing motor activity. The patient may show slowness and loss of dexterity, as well as problems with speech, manual skills, and gait.

Tremor is seen at rest and usually disappears when the affected limb is moved.

Rigidity is due to an abnormal increase in muscle tone, producing cogwheel resistance to passive movement of an extremity.

In addition, the patient may suffer from a stoop when standing or walking and a characteristic posturing of the hands and feet. Perspiration, excessive salivation, seborrhea, and difficulty in swallowing may also be seen.

ETIOLOGY OF PARKINSONISM

Role of Acetylcholine and Dopamine in the Basal Ganglia

The basal ganglia area of the brain is responsible for the smooth control of skeletal muscle movement. It contains high concentrations of the neurotransmitters acetylcholine (ACh) and dopamine (DA). The two appear to function as physiologic antagonists, with DA acting as an inhibitory neurotransmitter and ACh as an excitatory neurotransmitter. Normal control

203

of muscle movements depends on a delicate balance between these two. In patients with parkinsonism, this balance is destroyed, as the levels of DA in the basal ganglia are reduced and ACh acts unopposed. Figure 24–1 presents the concentrations of DA in the caudate nucleus and putamen areas of the basal ganglia. The depletion of DA can be correlated with the degree of degeneration of the substantia nigra. In the presence of a DA deficiency, the

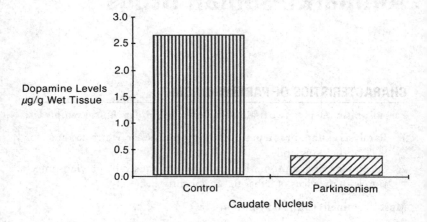

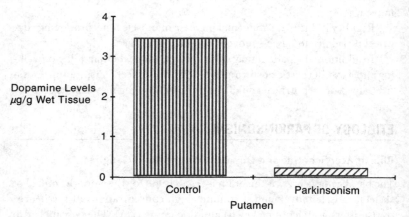

Figure 24–1 Concentrations of dopamine in the caudate nucleus and putamen at autopsy from controls and patients afflicted with parkinsonism. (After data provided in Hornykiewicz O. Parkinson's disease: from brain homogenates to treatment. Fed Proc 1973; 32:183–190.)

normal balance between DA and ACh is disturbed, and cholinergic activity predominates (Figure 24–2).

DRUGS FOR THE TREATMENT OF PARKINSONISM

Given the decreased levels of DA in the basal ganglia of parkinsonian patients, and the resulting cholinergic predominance, drug therapy is aimed at

A. stimulating DA receptors, and/or
B. blocking the cholinergic receptors in the basal ganglia.

1. Dopaminergic Drugs

A. Levodopa

Actions and Pharmacokinetics

Levodopa is the immediate precursor of DA. When administered, a small portion of levodopa enters the brain and is converted to DA by the enzyme dopa decarboxylase (refer to Chapter 3 for a review of dopamine synthesis). DA itself cannot be administered for the treatment of parkinsonism, because it will not cross the blood-brain barrier.

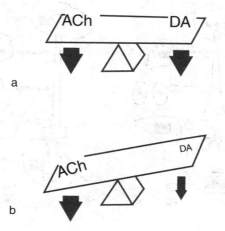

Figure 24–2 Diagrammatic representation of the balance between dopaminergic and cholinergic mechanisms in the striatum. ACh = acetylcholine; DA = dopamine; A = normal state; B = parkinsonism. (After Yahr MD. The treatment of parkinsonism. Med Clin North Am 1972; 56:1377–1382.)

Orally administered levodopa is extensively metabolized in peripheral tissues, with only a very small percentage being converted to DA in the brain (Figure 24–3). As a result, very large doses of the drug must be administered orally, accounting for the high incidence of levodopa-associated adverse effects.

Uses

Levodopa, alone or in combination with a dopa decarboxylase inhibitor, is the most useful drug for the treatment of Parkinson's disease. Although treatment may be started with an anticholinergic or amantadine, the disease usually progresses to the point where levodopa is required within one year.

The combination of levodopa and an anticholinergic may benefit patients who are not adequately treated by either drug alone.

Levodopa is contraindicated in patients with parkinsonism secondary to the use of antipsychotic drugs because it will reverse the therapeutic benefits provided by phenothiazines and butyrophenones (see Chapter 20).

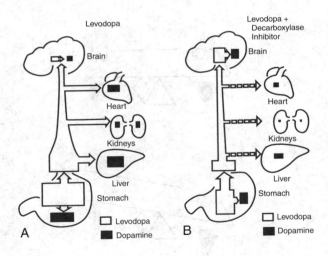

Figure 24–3 Diagrammatic representation of the peripheral decarboxylation of levodopa to dopamine (A) and the inhibition of this by the administration of a decarboxylase inhibitor (B). The concurrent administration of levodopa and a decarboxylase inhibitor decreases the amount of levodopa required to elicit a therapeutic response in parkinsonism. (After Selby G. Treatment of parkinsonism. Drugs 1976; 11:65.)

Adverse Effects

Levodopa can produce anorexia, nausea, vomiting, or epigastric pain. It may also produce mild postural hypotension and cardiac arrhythmias. Abnormal involuntary movements (faciolingual tics, grimacing, head bobbing, and various rocking and rotating movements of the arms, legs, or trunk) may also occur. Given to parkinsonian patients with impaired memory or dementia, levodopa can stimulate the CNS, resulting in hallucinations, paranoia, mania, insomnia, and nightmares. It can also cause depression. Levodopa can also stimulate the sexual interests of elderly patients.

B. Levodopa plus a Dopa Decarboxylase Inhibitor (Carbidopa or Benserazide)

Actions and Pharmacokinetics

Carbidopa and benserazide inhibit dopa decarboxylase. Because they do not cross the blood-brain barrier, these drugs reduce only the peripheral metabolism of levodopa to DA (see Figure 24–3). The formation of dopamine in the brain is not affected and a higher percentage of the administered levodopa is converted to DA in the brain. By using carbidopa or benserazide, it is possible to administer lower doses of levodopa, thereby reducing its peripheral adverse effects.

Uses and Adverse Effects

Products containing levodopa plus carbidopa and levodopa plus benserazide have replaced levodopa alone as the most useful treatment for parkinsonism. Because these products contain lower doses of levodopa, the incidence and severity of levodopa-induced adverse effects are reduced.

C. Levodopa/Dopa Decarboxylase Inhibitor, plus a Catechol-O-Methyltransferase Inhibitor (Entacapone)

Actions

Entacapone is a reversible, specific, and mainly peripherally acting inhibitor of catechol-*O*-methyltransferase (COMT) (see Chapter 3). COMT is responsible for the *O*-methylation of levodopa. In the presence of a dopa decarboxylase inhibitor, COMT becomes the major enzyme responsible for the peripheral metabolism of levodopa, converting it to the inactive 3-methoxy-4-hydroxy-l-phenylalanine (3-OMD). When administered with levodopa and a dopa decarboxylase inhibitor, entacapone further decreases the degradation of levodopa in the peripheral tissues. The ensuing sustained plasma levels of levodopa result in more constant dopaminergic stimulation in the brain, further reducing the signs and symptoms of Parkinson's disease.

Uses

Entacapone is used as an adjunct to a levodopa/dopa decarboxylase inhibitor for the treatment of the signs and symptoms of Parkinson's disease.

Adverse Effects

The most common adverse reaction to entacapone is diarrhea. Other adverse effects include dyskinesia, abdominal pain, and nausea.

D. Direct Dopamine Agonist (Bromocriptine)

Actions and Uses

Bromocriptine directly stimulates brain dopamine D_2-receptors. It is clinically useful as an adjunct to levodopa plus a dopa decarboxylase inhibitor in the symptomatic management of selected patients with Parkinson's disease who experience dyskinesia or "wearing-off" reactions on long-term levodopa therapy.

Adverse Effects

Bromocriptine's adverse effects include nausea, vomiting, transient dizziness, abdominal pain, constipation, and blurred vision, with or without diplopia. Digital vasospasm in response to cold, erythromelalgia, mental disturbances, and dyskinesias may also be experienced. In higher doses, bromocriptine can produce mental disturbance, including nightmares, mild agitation, hallucinations, and paranoid delusions. These are more common in the elderly.

E. Selective Monoamine Oxidase Type B (MAO-B) Inhibitor (Selegiline)

Actions

Selegiline may act by inhibiting MAO-B in the brain to reduce dopamine metabolism and increase the amount of DA available to stimulate brain receptors. Selegiline may also block DA neuronal uptake and this effect would also increase the amount of dopamine available to stimulate receptors.

Uses

Selegiline may be of value as an adjunct to levodopa (with or without a dopa decarboxylase inhibitor) in the management of the signs and symptoms of Parkinson's disease.

Adverse Effects

The adverse effects of recommended doses of selegiline are those usually associated with an excess of DA (see levodopa above). Hallucinations and confusion have been seen with the combined use of selegiline and levodopa/carbidopa. Other adverse effects include nausea, depression, loss of balance, insomnia, orthostatic hypotension, increased akinetic involuntary movements, arrhythmia, bradykinesia, involuntary movements, chorea, delusions, hypertension, angina, and syncope.

F. Dopamine-Releasing Drug (Amantadine)

Actions

Amantadine releases DA from the remaining intact dopaminergic nerves in the basal ganglia. Although less effective than levodopa, amantadine produces a more rapid response and fewer adverse effects.

Uses

Amantadine is indicated for the treatment of Parkinson's syndrome. Unfortunately, the initial clinical improvements may not be sustained. Performance deteriorates over 3 to 6 months. Therefore, amantadine is used most often in combination with levodopa as it often improves the effects of the latter.

Amantadine is also used in the short-term management of drug-induced extrapyramidal symptoms.

Adverse Effects

The more important adverse effects with amantadine are orthostatic hypotensive episodes, congestive heart failure, depression, psychosis, and urinary retention.

2. Central Anticholinergic Drugs (see Chapter 5) (Trihexyphenidyl HCl, Benztropine Mesylate, Procyclidine HCl, Biperiden HCl)

Actions and Uses

These drugs block central cholinergic receptors and reduce excessive cholinergic stimulation in basal ganglia. Classic anticholinergics, such as atropine and hyoscine, also block cholinergic receptors in the brain. However, their profound peripheral adverse effects prevent them from being used to treat parkinsonism. In contrast, the centrally acting anticholinergics have reduced peripheral effects, and accordingly decreased adverse effects. Central anticholinergic drugs are used in patients at the early stage of disease, for those with minor symptoms and in individuals who cannot tolerate levodopa. They are also used in combination with levodopa. Central anticholinergics are also used to reduce drug-induced parkinsonism (see Chapter 20).

Adverse Effects

The adverse effects of these drugs can mainly be attributed to a reduction in peripheral cholinergic stimulation (see Chapter 5). Although more selective than atropine, these drugs can still produce cycloplegia, urinary retention, and constipation. Because of their mydriatic effects, they can precipitate an attack of acute-angle glaucoma in patients predisposed to angle closure. The decrease in salivation that accompanies their use benefits the patient who experiences sialorrhea. Confusion and excitement can occur with large doses or in susceptible patients, such as elderly patients with existing mental disorders and those taking other drugs with anticholinergic properties. Care must be taken in using anticholinergic drugs in patients over the age of 70 or any individual with dementia.

Analgesics

NARCOTIC ANALGESICS (OPIOIDS)

General Properties of Narcotic Analgesics

Narcotic Receptors and the Mechanism of Action of Narcotic Analgesics

Opioids exert their analgesic activity by stimulating endogenous opioid receptors. An excellent correlation exists between the in vivo potencies of opioids and their in vitro affinities for opioid receptor binding sites. The three major classes of opioid receptors in the CNS are:

1. μ (mu). Morphine, its congeners, and endogenous opioid peptides produce supraspinal analgesia and euphoria by acting at μ_1-receptors, which are localized at the anatomic sites important for pain. The μ_2-receptors, appear to be involved in the production of respiratory depression and constipation. Narcotics also produce analgesia after intrathecal or epidural administration. This analgesia is mediated by an action at spinal μ-receptors.
2. κ (kappa) and δ (delta). The analgesic effects of both endogenous and synthetic peptides are mediated by these receptors. In addition, opioid agonist-antagonist analgesics, such as pentazocine, nalbuphine, and butorphanol, relieve pain and cause sedation by acting on κ-receptors. The dysphoric and psychotomimetic-like side effects observed after higher doses of these drugs are produced by an action at δ-receptors.

Effects Common to Narcotic Analgesics

Most narcotic analgesics share common pharmacologic properties. These are:

- **Euphoria** must not be minimized because the analgesia produced by narcotics depends to a great extent on the ability of narcotics to induce a sense of well-being.
- **Drowsiness** is a characteristic feature of stronger narcotics and plays a role in their analgesic effects.
- **Respiratory depression** occurs with even small doses, because narcotics reduce the sensitivity of the brain stem respiratory centers to increases in carbon dioxide (CO_2) tension.
- **Nausea and vomiting** may occur because narcotics stimulate the chemoreceptor trigger zone in the medulla of the brain.
- **Miosis** results from a stimulation of the autonomic segment of the nucleus of the oculomotor nerve.
- **Constipation** occurs with most narcotics. This is due to
  1. a delayed emptying of the stomach as a result of constriction of the pyloric sphincter and increased tone of the antral portion of the stomach and duodenum;
  2. a decrease in the propulsive contractions of the small intestine, together with an increase in nonpropulsive contractions and an increase in the tone of the colon; and
  3. an increase in the tone of the anal sphincter.
- **Increased biliary tract pressure** occurs with most narcotics. The symptoms range from epigastric distress to typical biliary colic.
- **Physiologic and psychological dependence** develop during chronic administration. If a dependent subject is suddenly deprived of a narcotic, physical withdrawal occurs quickly. The signs of physical withdrawal include autonomic hyperactivity, such as diarrhea, vomiting, lacrimation, rhinorrhea, chills, and fever. Individuals may also suffer from abdominal cramps, pain, and tremors. Psychological dependence is evident when an individual who has been weaned off a narcotic still feels a compulsion to take the drug.
- **Tolerance** occurs to the analgesic, euphoric, and respiratory-depressant effects of narcotics. If a narcotic is used daily over a prolonged period of time, larger and larger doses must be given to maintain the same degree of analgesia. Once a patient develops tolerance to one narcotic, he or she will show tolerance to all other narcotics (**cross-tolerance**).

Pharmacokinetics

Narcotics are usually well absorbed from the GI tract, but they are often extensively inactivated during their first pass through the liver (first-pass effect). As a result, the oral dose of a narcotic is usually larger than the parenteral dose. Most narcotics are effective for 3 to 5 hours.

Uses

The uses of narcotics include the treatment of:

- severe pain, resulting from trauma, surgery, obstetrics, renal biliary colic, and carcinoma;
- dyspnea, produced by left-ventricular failure and pulmonary failure. Because narcotics dilate veins, they reduce preload on the heart, thereby decreasing dyspnea;
- diarrhea. Loperamide is the preferred narcotic because it is very poorly absorbed; and
- cough. Narcotics depress the cough center in the medulla of the brain. Codeine and hydrocodone are most frequently used.

Adverse Effects

The major adverse effects of narcotic analgesics are respiratory depression, dependence, constipation, nausea, and vomiting. Because narcotics cause hypoventilation and hypercapnia, they dilate cerebral blood vessels and increase intracranial pressure. As a result, narcotics must be used very cautiously, if at all, in patients with head injuries, delirium tremens, and conditions in which intracranial pressure is increased.

Narcotics can cause hypotension and shock and they should be given in lower doses, if at all, to patients in shock or those with decreased blood volume.

The spasmogenic effect of narcotics on the urinary bladder can lead to urinary retention in patients with prostatic hypertrophy or urethral stricture.

Agonist-Antagonist Narcotic Analgesics

Actions, Uses, and Adverse Effects

Pentazocine, nalbuphine, and butorphanol are called agonist-antagonist narcotics. In the presence of a narcotic agonist, they block many of the actions of the narcotic. In the absence of a narcotic agonist, the agonist-antagonist drugs produce analgesia. This action can be explained by the fact that agonist-antagonist narcotics block μ-receptors, but stimulate κ-receptors. These drugs are used to relieve pain in the same manner as the other narcotics. Because they block μ-receptors, agonist-antagonist narcotics must not be administered to patients currently receiving an agonist narcotic. These drugs have the same general adverse effects as narcotics. Particular attention should be paid to the psychotomimetic effects of large doses of pentazocine. See Table 25–1.

Table 25–1
Examples of Narcotic and Agonist-Antagonist Narcotic Drugs

Drug	Comments
Agonist Narcotics	
Morphine	Prototype of strong analgesics. Relieves severe pain. Given orally or parenterally
Oxymorphone	Administered by IV or rectally for moderate to severe pain
Codeine	Used orally for mild to moderate pain, often with non-narcotic analgesics
Oxycodone	Used with non-narcotic analgesics for moderate to severe pain
Levorphanol	Used orally or parenterally for severe pain.
Meperidine	Used orally or parenterally for moderate to severe pain
Propoxyphene	Used orally, often with non-narcotic analgesics, for mild to moderate pain
Fentanyl, Sufentanil, Alfentanil, and Remifentanil	Administered by IV, for pain relief during surgery
Agonist-Antagonist Narcotics	
Pentazocine	Given orally or parenterally for moderate pain
Butorphanol	Given parenterally for moderate to severe pain
Nalbuphine	Given parenterally for moderate to severe pain

IV = intravenous

NARCOTIC ANTAGONISTS (NALOXONE)

Actions, Uses and Adverse Effects

Narcotic antagonists, such as naloxone, competitively block opiate receptors. They produce few effects in patients who have not been treated with an opioid, however, in patients previously treated with a narcotic, naxolone reverses the effects of the narcotic. Narcotic antagonists are used to treat narcotic overdoses or reverse the effects of a narcotic given during surgery. Abrupt withdrawal of narcotic depression may result in nausea, vomiting, sweating, tachycardia, increased BP, and tremors.

NON-NARCOTIC ANALGESICS (ANALGESIC-ANTIPYRETICS)

1. Acetylsalicylic Acid (ASA) (Aspirin)

Actions (for the Antiplatelet and Antiarthritic Actions of ASA, Refer to Chapters 15 and 26)

Analgesia Aspirin works both peripherally and within the brain to produce analgesia. Peripherally, aspirin inhibits cyclooxygenase to reduce the formation of prostaglandin E_2 (PGE_2) in various organs and tissues (Figure 25–1). PGE_2 sensitizes pain receptors to noxious substances, such as histamine and bradykinin. By reducing the synthesis of PGE_2, aspirin diminishes pain. Centrally, the drug acts in the hypothalamus to reduce pain perception. Since aspirin does not affect the cortex of the brain, analgesic doses do not cause mental disturbance or drowsiness.

 Antipyresis Therapeutic doses of aspirin lower elevated body temperatures. Toxic doses increase temperature. The antipyretic effects are due to

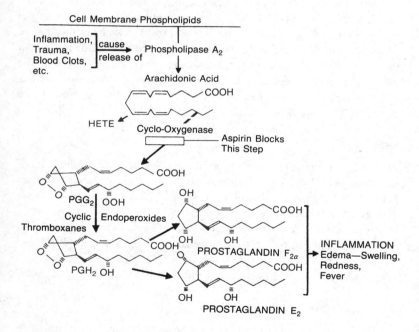

Figure 25–1 Inhibition of prostaglandin synthesis by aspirin. PG = prostaglandin; HETE = hydroxyeicosatetaraenoic acid (After Mazel P. Analgesics-antipyretics. In: Pradhan SN, Maickel RP, Dutta SN, ed. Pharmacology in Medicine. Bethesda, MD: SP Press International, 1986:224.)

aspirin's action on the hypothalamus in the brain. In normal individuals, the hypothalamus maintains body temperature within narrow limits by balancing heat production with heat loss. Aspirin lowers elevated temperature by several means. In a person with a fever, aspirin dilates small blood vessels in the skin, thereby increasing heat loss by sweating. It also prevents the temperature-elevating effects of leukocytic pyrogens, possibly by competing with pyrogens for receptor sites in the thermoregulatory centers of the hypothalamus. Fever typically occurs from a disease state that increases cytokine production. Cytokines, such interleukin-1 (IL-1) and tumor necrosis factor, stimulate the synthesis of PGE_2, which in turn increases body temperature. Because aspirin inhibits cyclooxygenase, it may owe some of the antipyretic effects to the resulting decrease in PGE_2 synthesis.

Pharmacokinetics

Aspirin can be absorbed from the stomach, but its absorption proceeds faster from the duodenum. Shortly after its absorption, aspirin is metabolized to salicylic acid. Salicylic acid is then metabolized mainly in the liver to salicylic acyl glucuronide, salicylic phenol glucuronide, salicyluric acid, and gentisic acid (Figure 25–2). Salicyluric acid, a glycine conjugate, accounts for 75% of the metabolites. The capacity of the liver to furnish enough glycine to inactivate salicylate is limited. If the daily dose of aspirin exceeds the capacity of the liver to provide glycine, serum salicylate levels rise sharply and the patient may become toxic. About 10% of the salicylate in the body is eliminated unchanged by the kidney. If the urine is alkalinized, this can be increased 3- to 5-fold.

Uses

Aspirin is an effective analgesic and antipyretic for the relief of mild to moderate pain. Aspirin is more effective in the relief of skeletal muscle pain than visceral pain and is often given to patients with headaches, neuralgias, myalgias, or primary spasmodic dysmenorrhea.

   Because of concern over a possible correlation between the use of ASA as an antipyretic in children with varicella or influenza virus infection and the development of Reye's syndrome authorities advise that ASA not be used in children, teenagers, or young adults with varicella or influenza.

Adverse Effects

Gastric irritation, ranging from discomfort to gastric ulceration and hemorrhage, is a common adverse effect of aspirin due to

- its direct irritant effects on the gastric mucosa, and

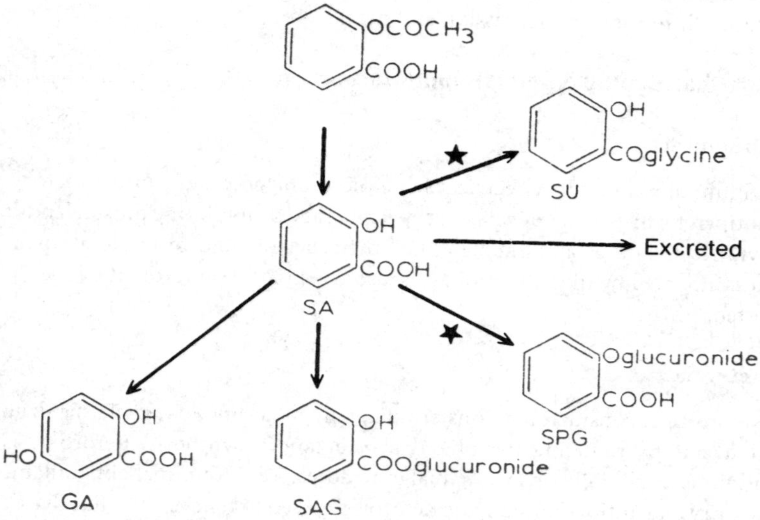

Figure 25–2 Metabolism of acetylsalicylic acid. * = 2 processes which proceed by easily saturable Michaelis-Menten kinetics. ASA – acetylsalicylic acid, SA – salicylic acid, GA – gentisic acid, SAG – salicylic acyl glucuronide, SPG – salicylic phenol glucuronide, SU – salicyluric acid. (After Thiessen JJ. Pharmacokinetics of salicylates. In: Barnett HJM, Hirsch J, Mustard JF, eds. Acetylsalicylic acid, new uses for an old drug. New York: Raven Press, 1982:53.)

- its ability to inhibit prostaglandin formation. PGE_2 promotes the secretion of protective gastric mucus. When its formation is blocked by ASA, the secretion of mucous in the stomach falls and gastric damage occurs.

Enteric-coated tablets prevent the direct irritant effect of aspirin on the gastric mucosa. However, enteric coating has no effect on the ability of aspirin, delivered back to the stomach in the circulation, to inhibit cyclooxygenase and inhibit the formation of prostaglandins.

Hypoprothrombinemia can be produced by large doses of aspirin because salicylate is a vitamin K antagonist. This effect is usually only significant in patients taking oral anticoagulants or suffering from liver disease.

Serious allergic reactions, including asthmatic attacks, can occur from ASA use. Patients allergic to aspirin should not be given any nonsteroidal anti-inflammatory drug (NSAID).

Large doses of aspirin can be very toxic. Beginning with tinnitus and decreased hearing, the symptoms of acute poisoning can proceed to respiratory alkalosis. In response to the increased loss of CO_2, renal excretion of bicarbonate rises and systemic pH returns to normal, but at the cost of a reduced bicarbonate reserve. If sufficient ASA is consumed, metabolic rate increases and metabolic acidosis ensues. The final stage in salicylate intoxication is respiratory depression and death.

2. Other Cyclooxygenase Inhibitors

Diflunisal

Diflunisal is an orally effective nonsteroidal, analgesic, anti-inflammatory, antipyretic drug that appears to act peripherally by inhibiting prostaglandin synthesis. Diflunisal is indicated for the relief of mild to moderate pain accompanied by inflammation. It is also used in the symptomatic relief of osteoarthritis.

Ketorolac

Ketorolac is considered a nonsteroidal, anti-inflammatory, analgesic drug that acts by reducing peripheral prostaglandin synthesis. Ketorolac is administered orally or IM. At analgesic doses, it has minimal anti-inflammatory and antipyretic activity. Ketorolac is used to relieve pain. Its adverse effects are similar to those of the other NSAIDs (see Chapter 26) and include dyspepsia and GI pain.

Nonsteroidal Anti-inflammatory Drugs (see Chapter 26)

Like aspirin, NSAIDs inhibit the formation of the various prostaglandins. As a result, NSAIDs can be used as analgesic-antipyretics. Drugs such as ibuprofen, naproxen sodium, and fenoprofen are sold as analgesics. They are effective in mild to moderate pain. Their pharmacology and adverse effects are presented in Chapter 26.

3. Acetaminophen, Paracetamol

Actions

Acetaminophen is an analgesic and antipyretic. It does not have the anti-inflammatory effects of aspirin. Acetaminophen does not affect platelet aggregation or irritate the stomach.

Uses

Acetaminophen is indicated for the treatment of mild to moderate pain and for the reduction of fever. The major use for the drug is as an analgesic-antipyretic in patients who cannot tolerate aspirin (eg, patients who suffer GI discomfort or are allergic to ASA). Acetaminophen should also be used in place of aspirin in patients taking oral anticoagulants.

The drug is also valuable in relieving the pain of osteoarthritis.

The connection between the use of ASA in children with varicella or influenza virus infection and the development of Reye's syndrome has led to the recommendation that acetaminophen, rather than ASA, be used in these conditions.

Adverse Effects

Taken in recommended doses, acetaminophen is well tolerated. Hepatic necrosis can occur if overdoses are taken. This toxicity results from a change in the normal pathway of acetaminophen metabolism, which occurs with high doses of the drug. Approximately 25% percent of the absorbed dose of acetaminophen undergoes first-pass metabolism. The major metabolites are sulfate and glucuronide conjugates (Figure 25–3). If large doses (10 to 15 g) are taken, the capacity of the liver to form sulfate and glucuronide conjugates is exceeded. When this happens, acetaminophen undergoes N-hydroxylation to form *N*-acetyl-benzoquinoneimine, a highly reactive intermediate. This metabolite reacts with sulfhydryl groups in proteins and glutathione. When hepatic glutathione is depleted by very large doses of acetaminophen, reaction of this metabolite with hepatic proteins is increased and liver necrosis occurs.

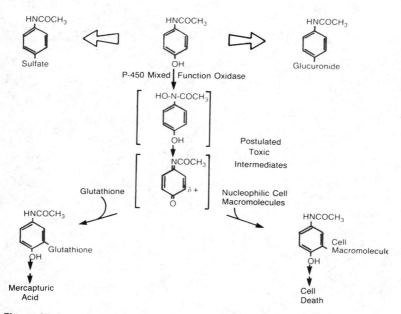

Figure 25–3 Pathways of acetaminophen metabolism. (After Mitchell JR, et al. Acetaminophen-induced hepatic injury: protective role of glutathione in man and rationale for therapy. Clin Pharm Therap 1974; 16:676–684.)

Treatment of acetaminophen overdosage includes

1. gavaging the patient or inducing vomiting, and
2. administering N-acetylcysteine. This compound appears to protect the liver by replenishing the stores of glutathione.

26

Antiarthritic and Antigout Drugs

ANTIARTHRITIC DRUGS

1. First-Line Drugs

A. Nonsteroidal Anti-inflammatory Drugs (NSAIDs) – Acetylsalicylic Acid (ASA) (Aspirin), Diclofenac, Fenoprofen, Flurbiprofen, Ibuprofen, Indomethacin, Ketoprofen, Naproxen, Piroxicam, Sulindac, Tiaprofenic Acid, Tolmetin

Actions (see Figure 25–1)

NSAIDs inhibit cyclooxygenase, thereby reducing prostaglandin synthesis. Specifically, they reduce the synthesis of prostaglandins PGE_2 and $PGF_{2\alpha}$. These chemicals increase the activities of two endogenous mediators of inflammation, histamine and bradykinin. In the face of reduced levels of PGE_2 and $PGF_{2\alpha}$, the ability of histamine and bradykinin to dilate blood vessels, increase vascular permeability, and produce pain is reduced. Other effects of NSAIDs that depend on their ability to inhibit prostaglandin formation include:

- **Analgesia** — PGE_2 and $PGF_{2\alpha}$ sensitize nerve endings to pain.
- **Antipyresis** — NSAIDs lower elevated body temperatures by dilating the small vessels in the skin of the patient with a fever and increasing heat loss. NSAIDs may also reduce heat production by reducing prostaglandin formation in the hypothalamus. Prostaglandins are necessary for pyrogen-induced fever.
- **Gastric irritation** — NSAIDs irritate the stomach directly. They can also damage the stomach after they are absorbed, due to an inhibition

of PGE_2 and PGI_2 synthesis in the gastric mucosa. PGE_2 and PGI_2 inhibit gastric acid secretion and promote the secretion of cytoprotective mucus in the intestine. By blocking the production of PGE_2 and PGI_2, NSAIDs predispose the stomach to ulceration.

- **Reduce platelet aggregation** — Some NSAIDs inhibit platelet aggregation (see Chapter 15).
- **Decreased renal function** — PGE_2 increases the renal excretion of sodium, chloride, and water. Inhibition of its formation results in salt and water reabsorption. Renal prostaglandins reduce the vasoconstriction produced by norepinephrine and angiotensin II. In patients with reduced renal function, prostaglandins are important in maintaining renal flow. In these patients, NSAIDs can significantly reduce renal function.

Uses

NSAIDs are used to provide relief from the symptoms of rheumatoid arthritis, osteoarthritis, spondylitis, bursitis, and other forms of rheumatism and musculoskeletal disorders.

NSAIDs are also used as analgesics (see Chapter 25).

Adverse Effects

NSAIDs can produce nausea, vomiting, diarrhea, gastritis, GI bleeding and/or ulceration, tinnitus, vertigo, hearing loss, leukopenia, thrombocytopenia, purpura, urticaria, and angioedema.

They can also cause pruritus and skin eruptions, asthma, anaphylaxis, reversible hepatotoxicity, mental confusion, drowsiness, sweating, and thirst.

B. Cyclooxygenase-2 (COX-2) Inhibitors (Celecoxib and Rofecoxib)

Actions, Uses, and Adverse Effects

Two forms of cyclooxygenase exist (COX-1 and COX-2). COX-1 is constitutively expressed and enzymatically active in various tissues, including the stomach, intestines, kidneys, and also in platelets. COX-1 is responsible for prostaglandin-mediated normal physiologic functions such as cytoprotection and platelet aggregation, and is involved in renal function. Inhibition of COX-1 has been associated with gastric damage and renal toxicity. COX-2 is the inducible isoform of the enzyme that has been shown to be up-regulated by proinflammatory stimuli. COX-2 has been postulated to be primarily responsible for the synthesis of the prostanoid mediators of pain, inflammation, and fever.

NSAIDs inhibit both COX-1 and COX-2. Therapeutic concentrations of COX-2 inhibitors (celecoxib and rofecoxib) do not significantly inhibit COX-1. These drugs produce their anti-inflammatory effects by inhibiting COX-2, but because they do not significantly inhibit COX-1, they do not produce the frequently severe gastric damage produced by NSAIDs.

2. Second-Line Drugs

A. Antimalarial Drugs (Chloroquine and Hydroxychloroquine)

Actions, Uses, and Adverse Effects

Although their mechanism of action is not understood, both chloroquine phosphate and hydroxychloroquine sulfate are used for rheumatoid arthritis, juvenile arthritis, and for the arthritic and skin manifestations of systemic lupus erythematosus.

The most common adverse effect is eye damage. This may involve

(1) corneal infiltration, which is reversible on stopping the drug, or
(2) retinopathy, which can lead to irreversible visual loss.

These drugs may also cause gastric intolerance.

B. Gold Compounds (Aurothioglucose and Gold Sodium Thiomalate — Administered Parenterally) (Auranofin — Administered Orally)

Actions, Uses, and Adverse Effects

Gold's mechanism of action is not known. Gold has a delayed onset of action. Treatment must be continued for at least a few months. These drugs are useful and may even alter the course of arthritis in patients with adult or juvenile rheumatoid arthritis, or psoriatic arthritis.

Gold compounds may produce rash, mucous membrane lesions, serious hematologic complications, and proteinuria. Auranofin can also cause GI disturbances.

C. Penicillamine

Actions, Uses and Adverse Effects

Penicillamine may have an immunosuppressive action on T cells. It is as effective as gold or azathioprine in treating rheumatoid arthritis but of little value in ankylosing spondylitis or psoriatic arthritis. Skin rashes and GI disturbances are the most common adverse effects, but renal damage or bone marrow depression are the major reasons for stopping the drug.

D. Azathioprine

Actions, Uses, and Adverse Effects

Azathioprine is an immunosuppressant that should be used only in severe, active, progressive rheumatoid arthritis that has failed to respond to conventional treatment. It should be given with NSAIDs; however, gold, antimalarials, and penicillamine should be stopped.

Azathioprine can cause nausea and vomiting, leukopenia, thrombocytopenia, and anemia. Complete blood counts, including platelet counts, should be performed periodically.

E. Methotrexate

Actions, Uses, and Adverse Effects

Methotrexate is a competitive inhibitor of folic acid reductase, but its mechanism of action in rheumatoid arthritis is unknown. Usually, the effects of methotrexate on articular swelling and tenderness in rheumatoid arthritis can be seen as early as 3 to 6 weeks. It is indicated in the management of selected adults with severe, active, or definite rheumatoid arthritis who have an insufficient response to, or were intolerant of, an adequate trial of first-line therapy and usually a trial of a least one or more disease-modifying antirheumatic drugs as well.

The most common adverse effects include nausea, stomatitis, GI discomfort, diarrhea, vomiting, and anorexia. Laboratory findings include elevation of liver enzymes and, occasionally, decreased WBC.

F. Adrenal Corticosteroids

Uses (see Chapter 18 for Actions and Adverse Effects)

Corticosteroids may be administered systemically when more conservative measures fail or during the hiatus between the initiation of second-line therapy and its onset of action in a patient whose condition cannot be controlled by rest, physical measures, analgesics, and NSAIDs.

Intra-articular therapy may be indicated for

1. the patient with otherwise well-controlled arthritis in whom a single joint is particularly resistant,
2. the individual in whom one or two particularly active joints flare and impede ambulation or physiotherapy, or
3. the patient with one active joint, in whom NSAIDs are contraindicated.

G. Infliximab

Actions

Although the precise pathophysiology of rheumatoid arthritis (RA) remains to be elucidated, it is believed to involve a T-cell-mediated immune response that results in the release of the cytokines interleukin-1 (IL-1) and tumor necrosis factor alpha (TNF_α). Infliximab is a recombinant chimeric human-murine IgG_κ monoclonal antibody that neutralizes TNF_α in the joints of RA patients by binding specifically to both soluble and transmembrane TNF_α.

Uses

When added to methotrexate therapy, infliximab reduces the signs and symptoms of moderate to severe rheumatoid arthritis. Infliximab appears to be the only therapy, to date, that is effective in arresting and potentially reversing the structural damage seen in severe RA patients.

Adverse Effects

From information to date, infliximab appears to be a safe medication. The adverse effect profile is similar to that of placebo.

ANTIGOUT DRUGS

Etiology of Gout

Gout is a disorder of uric acid metabolism. The normal range for serum urate concentrations is 3 to 8 mg/100 mL (190–490 mmol/L). People with serum urate concentrations in this range have little risk of gout. Individuals at high risk have serum urate levels of 10 to 11 mg/100mL (610–675 mmol/L). These concentrations exceed the capacity of the blood fluids to hold urate in solution, and, therefore, sodium urate crystals may deposit in a joint. When neutrophils attempt to phagocytose the crystals, inflammation ensues and the patient experiences gout (Figure 26–1).

Mechanism of Action of Antigout Drugs

Antigout drugs can act

(1) in the joint to reduce inflammation,
(2) in the tissues to decrease the production of uric acid, or
(3) in the kidneys to increase uric acid excretion.

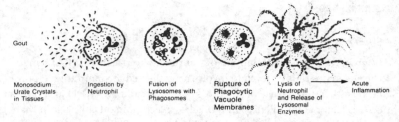

Figure 26–1 Role of monosodium urate crystals and neutrophils in gout. (After Ryan GB, Majno G. Inflammation. Kalamazoo, MI: Scope Productions. The Upjohn Co. 1974: 54.)

1. Drugs that Act in the Joint

A. Colchicine

Actions

Colchicine concentrates in neutrophils and decreases the release of chemo-tactic factors from the neutrophils, with the result that fewer neutrophils are subsequently attracted to the affected joint.

Uses

Colchicine is effective in relieving the pain of acute attacks of gout, especially if therapy is begun early in the attack.

During the initial treatment with allopurinol or uricosurics, patients often experience more attacks. Colchicine can be given at this time to reduce the number of attacks.

Adverse Effects

Diarrhea, nausea, vomiting, and abdominal pain often occur. Large doses can cause a burning sensation in the throat, bloody diarrhea, hematuria, oliguria, CNS depression, and death.

B. Nonsteroidal Anti-Inflammatory Drugs (NSAIDs)

Actions, Uses, and Adverse Effects

The actions and adverse effects of these drugs have been presented earlier in this chapter. NSAIDs have largely replaced colchicine for acute attacks because of colchicine's invariable tendency to produce GI upset. To be effective for gout, optimal doses of NSAIDs should be used promptly.

2. Drugs that Reduce Uric Acid Synthesis

Allopurinol

Actions and Uses

Allopurinol and its major metabolite, oxypurinol, inhibit xanthine oxidase, the enzyme response for the synthesis of uric acid. Both plasma and urine uric acid levels fall within a few days to two weeks of starting treatment. Allopurinol is used to treat chronic tophaceous gout.

Adverse Effects

Skin rashes, GI upset, hepatotoxicity, and fever are the most common adverse effects of allopurinol.

Attacks of acute gout may occur more frequently during the first months of treatment with allopurinol.

3. Drugs that Increase Renal Excretion of Uric Acid (Uricosurics)

Probenecid

Actions

Uric acid undergoes filtration, reabsorption, and secretion in the nephron as outlined below:

1. First, uric acid is filtered through the renal glomeruli.
2. Second, some of the filtered uric acid is reabsorbed back into the blood from the proximal convoluted tubules.
3. Finally, uric acid is secreted from the blood into the renal tubules.

The amount of uric acid cleared in the urine is the result of:

$$filtration + secretion - reabsorption$$

Probenecid decreases uric acid reabsorption. The resulting increase in uric acid excretion reduces its plasma level. However, even high doses of probenecid fail to prevent more than 50% of the filtered uric acid from being reabsorbed.

Uses

Probenecid is used to treat hyperuricemia in all stages of gout and gouty arthritis, except in an acute-presenting attack.

Adverse Effects

Probenecid's adverse effects include headache, anorexia, nausea, vomiting, urinary frequency, hypersensitivity reactions (dermatitis, pruritus, and fever), sore gums, flushing dizziness, anemia, and anaphylactoid reactions.

Hemolytic anemia has been reported. This may be related to a genetic glucose-6-phosphate dehydrogenase deficiency in red blood cells.

27

Antimigraine Drugs

Migraine headaches are caused by dilation of the arteries of the scalp, together with the release of 5-hydroxytryptamine (5-HT, serotonin), histamine, bradykinin, substance P, and prostaglandins that all sensitize pain receptors in the scalp vessel wall and adjoining tissue. Pulsation in the scalp arteries, together with sensitization of pain receptors, leads to the pain of migraine.

Rationale Behind Drug Therapy of Migraine Headaches

Drugs are used to:

1. prevent attacks (Note: The disparity in the mechanisms of action of drugs used to prevent migraine headaches (see below) reflects our lack of understanding of the multifactorial etiology of migraine headaches and our willingness to try many types of drugs in an attempt to prevent attacks.), and
2. terminate an attack, by producing analgesia or constricting the already dilated vessels.

1. Drugs to Prevent Migraine Attacks

A. Beta Blockers (Propranolol)

Actions, Uses, and Adverse Effects

Propranolol reduces the number of moderately severe migraine attacks in more than 50% of cases. Propranolol is often ineffective in patients with severe migraine. The adverse effects of propranolol were described in Chapter 6.

B. Tricyclic Antidepressants (TCAs) (Amitriptyline)

Actions, Uses, and Adverse Effects

TCAs (see Chapter 21) can prevent migraine in some patients and may be given concurrently with other prophylactic agents. Their mechanism of action in preventing migraine headaches is not clear. Amitriptyline has been used most frequently. It appears to be an effective prophylactic in about 55 to 60% of migraine patients.

C. 5-Hydroxytryptamine (5-HT) Antagonists

1. Pizotyline

Pizotyline blocks 5-HT receptors but it is not clear whether this mechanism explains the drug's ability to prevent migraine attacks. Approximately 33 to 66% of patients respond to the drug after 3 to 4 weeks of treatment. Its adverse effects include CNS depression, increase in appetite, and weight gain.

2. Methysergide

Methysergide is a 5-HT antagonist. It is not clear whether this action explains, or is just coincidental to, its ability to prevent migraine attacks. With a 70 to 80% success rate, methysergide is more effective than most other drugs, but it is also more toxic. Its adverse effects have limited its use to patients who do not respond to other drugs. Methysergide is indicated in the prophylactic treatment of severe recurring vascular headaches that occur at least once weekly, or in vascular headaches that are so severe or uncontrollable that preventative therapy is indicated regardless of frequency. Methysergide has proven effective in reducing or eliminating the pain and frequency of attacks of classic migraine, common migraine, and cluster headache (histaminic cephalgia).

Adverse Effects

Methysergide may produce retroperitoneal fibrosis as well as fibrosis in the pleura and heart valves. Because the risk of these adverse effects increases with the length of treatment, methysergide should not be taken continuously for longer than 6 months. Other adverse effects include insomnia, nausea, vomiting, heartburn, abdominal discomfort, and diarrhea.

D. Calcium Channel Blocker (Flunarizine)

Actions

Flunarizine is a calcium channel blocker that has no direct effects on the heart. Migraine pathogenesis likely involves an initial decrease in cerebral blood flow, leading to ischemia and hypoxia. Hypoxia, in turn, causes an excessive influx of calcium into cells resulting in cerebral cellular dysfunction. By blocking calcium entry channels, flunarizine

- inhibits the contraction of vascular smooth muscle mediated by the entry of extravascular calcium, and
- protects endothelial cells against damage from calcium overload and brain cells from hypoxia.

Uses

Flunarizine prevents migraine attacks at least as well as the other drugs discussed in this chapter. Flunarizine is most beneficial for reducing migraine frequency. It appears to have less effect on the severity and duration of attacks.

Adverse Effects

Flunarizine is usually well tolerated. Its adverse effects include depression, drowsiness, weight gain, headache, insomnia, nausea, gastric pain, and dry mouth.

E. Nonsteroidal Anti-Inflammatory Drugs (NSAIDs)

Actions, Uses, and Adverse Effects

The pharmacology of NSAIDs was presented in Chapter 26. These drugs are effective in both preventing and terminating migraine attacks.

2. Drugs to Treat Migraine Attacks

A. Analgesics

Actions, Uses, and Adverse Effects

Analgesics, such as aspirin with codeine, may relieve migraine pain. They are best taken early in the attack before pain has had an opportunity to become established. Narcotics stronger than codeine are not recommended because of the danger of dependence. NSAIDs can be quite effective in the treatment of migraine attacks. The pharmacology and adverse effects of these drugs were presented in Chapters 25 and 26.

B. Ergotamine and Dihydroergotamine

Actions

Ergotamine and dihydroergotamine are vasoconstrictors that reduce migraine-induced vasodilatation. They should not be used in patients with pre-existing vascular disease, such as atherosclerosis, hypertension, Raynaud's phenomenon, and Buerger's disease because of the risk of ischemia.

Uses

Ergotamine and dihydroergotamine abort migraine attacks. They should be taken as soon as the patient feels an attack starting.

Adverse Effects

The major adverse effects of these drugs are generalized vasoconstriction and stimulation of the vomiting center in the brain. Patients may experience nausea and vomiting, weakness in the legs, muscle pains in the extremities, numbness and tingling of fingers and toes, precordial distress and pain, and transient tachycardia or bradycardia.

C. 5-Hydroxytryptamine₁-Like Receptor Agonist (Sumatriptan)

Actions

Sumatriptan is a selective $5-HT_1$-like receptor agonist. The activation of $5-HT_1$ receptors located on intracranial blood vessels leads to vasoconstriction, which is believed to be correlated with the relief of migraine headaches.

Uses

Sumatriptan is indicated for the relief of migraine attacks, with or without aura. The drug is contraindicated in patients with ischemic heart disease, angina pectoris, previous myocardial infarction, and uncontrolled hypertension. Sumatriptan is also contraindicated in patients taking ergotamine-containing preparations.

Adverse Effects

The most common adverse effect of subcutaneous sumatriptan is transient pain at the site of injection. Other side effects of oral or subcutaneous sumatriptan include sensations of tingling, heat, heaviness, pressure or tightness in any part of the body, chest symptoms, flushing, dizziness, and feelings of weakness.

28

Beta-Lactam Antibiotics

PENICILLINS AND CEPHALOSPORINS

Actions (Figures 28–1 to 28–5)

Bacterial cells are encased by both cell membranes and cell walls. The cell wall lies on the outside of the bacterium and is essential to the survival of the microbe. Bacterial cytoplasm is hypertonic. Without a rigid cell wall, the cell membrane cannot withstand the internal hypertonic media. If the cell wall is damaged, the high pressure within the bacterium causes the membrane to first bulge and finally to rupture, killing the bacterium.

In forming a cell wall, adjacent peptidoglycan strands are cross-linked, giving the wall its strength. The transpeptidation reaction responsible for cross-linking involves cleavage of the terminal alanine from the pentapeptide attached to N-acetylglucosamine. A cross-link is formed between the lysine of one peptide chain to the first of the two D-alanines on another peptide chain.

Penicillins and cephalosporins are structurally similar to the terminal D-alanyl-D-alanine portion and, therefore, can compete for, and bind to, the enzyme that catalyzes transpeptidation and cross-linking. As the old walls gradually deteriorate and are not replaced by new material, they become thinner. Eventually, they are not strong enough to support the cell membranes, which then rupture, killing the bacteria.

THE PENICILLINS

Antibacterial Spectra

Tables 28–1 and 28–2 present the properties and antibacterial spectra of the three groups of penicillins.

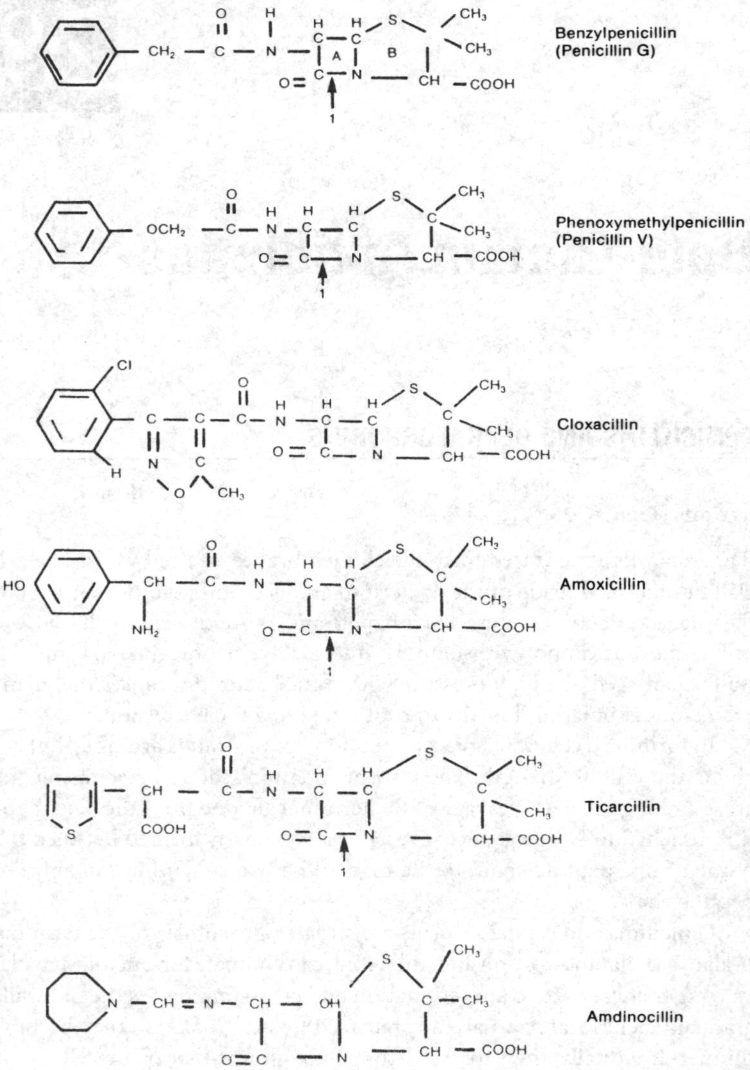

Figure 28–1 Structures of representative penicillins.

A = beta-lactam ring

B = thiazolidine ring

1 = site of action of penicillinase (beta-lactamase).

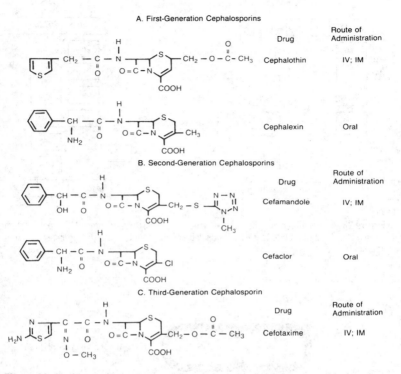

Figure 28–2 Structures of representative cephalosporins. IV = intravenous; IM = intramuscular.

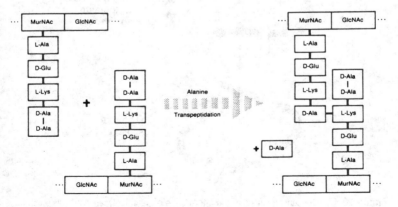

Figure 28–3 The chemical details of the transpeptidation reaction. (After Richmond MH. Beta-lactam antibiotics, the background to their use as therapeutic agents. Frankfurt: Hoechst Aktiegesellschaft; 1981.)

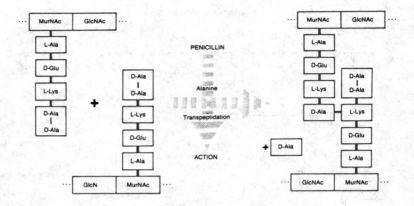

Figure 28–4 Inhibition of transpeptidation by penicillins. (After Richmond MH. Beta-lactam antibiotics, the background to their use as therapeutic agents. Frankfurt: Hoechst Aktiegesellschaft; 1981.)

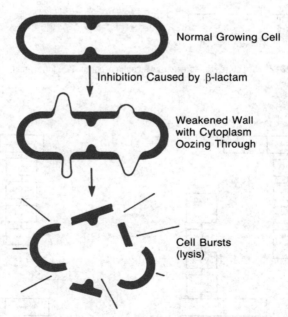

Figure 28–5 The consequences of the interruption of peptidoglycan synthesis, such as is caused by penicillins and cephalosporins. (After Richmond MH. Beta-lactam antibiotics, the background to their use as therapeutic agents. Frankfurt: Hoechst Aktiegesellschaft; 1981.)

Table 28–1
Properties of Some Commonly Used Penicillins

Type of Penicillin	Stability in Acid	Spectrum of Action	Sensitivity to Penicillinase	Admin. Routes
Narrow-spectrum penicillins				
Penicillin G (Benzylpenicillin)	Poor	Narrow	Sensitive	Oral and parenteral
Penicillin V (Phenoxymethyl penicillin)	Good	Narrow	Sensitive	Oral
Penicillinase-resistant penicillins				
Methicillin	Poor	Narrow	Resistant	Parenteral
Cloxacillin	Good	Narrow	Resistant	Oral and parenteral
Dicloxacillin	Good	Narrow	Resistant	Oral and parenteral
Flucloxacillin	Good	Narrow	Resistant	Oral
Expanded-Spectrum Penicillins				
Ampicillin	Fair	Broad	Sensitive	Oral and parenteral
Amoxicillin	Good	Broad	Sensitive	Oral
Ticarcillin	Poor	Broad	Sensitive	Parenteral
Piperacillin	Poor	Broad	Sensitive	Parenteral

1. Narrow-spectrum penicillins
2. Penicillinase-resistant penicillins
3. Expanded-spectrum penicillins

To understand the need for the different groups of penicillins, one must understand the limitations of penicillin G. Penicillin G:

1. is not stable in an acid media and is poorly absorbed from the GI tract,
2. is inactivated by penicillinase-producing staphylococci, and
3. has a narrow spectrum of activity.

To varying degrees, the newer penicillins overcome some of these shortcomings of penicillin G (see below).

Table 28–2
Antibacterial Spectra of the Various Penicillin Groups

	Narrow-Spectrum Penicillins		Expanded-Spectrum Penicillins	
	Penicillin G Penicillin V (Penicillinase-Sensitive Penicillins)	**Cloxacillin Dicloxacillin (Penicillinase-Resistant Penicillins)**	**Ampicillin Amoxicillin Bacampicillin Pivampicillin**	**Azlocillin Mezlocillin Piperacillin Ticarcillin**
Staphylococcus aureus (pen sensitive)	+	+	+	+
Staphylococcus aureus (pen resistant)	−	+	−	−
Streptococcus pyogenes	+	+	+	+
Streptococcus pneumoniae	+	+	+	+
Enterococcus spp.	−	−	+	−
Clostridium perfringens	+	+	+	+
Neisseria gonorrhoeae	+	±	+	+
Neisseria meningitidis	+	±	+	+
Haemophilus influenzae	−	−	±	+
Escherichia coli	−	−	±	±
Klebsiella spp.	−	−	−	±
Proteus spp. (indole negative)	−	−	±	+
Proteus spp. (indole positive)	−	−	−	±
Serratia spp.	−	−	−	±
Salmonella spp.	−	−	+	+
Shigella spp.	−	−	±	+
Pseudomonas aeruginosa	−	−	−	+
Bacteroides fragilis	−	−	−	±
Other *Bacteroides* spp.	+	±	+	±
Chlamydiae spp.	−	−	−	−
Mycobacteria pneumoniae	−	−	−	−

+ = sensitive;
− = resistant;
± = some strains resistant.

Pharmacokinetics of the Penicillins (Figure 28–6)

Absorption Most penicillins are destroyed, at least in part, by stomach acid. About two-thirds of an oral dose of penicillin G is destroyed by gastric acid, with only approximately one-third being absorbed. Penicillin G should be administered parenterally.

Parenterally, penicillin G is available in three forms, which differ in their absorption characteristics.

- Intramuscular (IM) penicillin G produces peak blood levels within 15 minutes.
- IM procaine penicillin G produces peak blood levels in 2 to 3 hours, with concentrations falling to 0 in 24 hours.
- IM benzathine penicillin G produces very low penicillin blood levels for 3 to 4 weeks.

Distribution All penicillins are distributed widely throughout the body. Their passage into joint, ocular, and cerebral spinal fluids (CSF) is poor in the absence of inflammation. In patients with inflamed meninges, however, they will enter the CSF.

Elimination All penicillins are rapidly excreted by renal tubular secretion, with renal clearance values of approximately 600 mL/min and half-lives of about 1 hour. Probenecid will reduce the renal tubular secretion of penicillins and prolong their half-lives.

Penicillin G

Penicillin G is preferred for infections caused by frequently encountered gram-positive bacteria and susceptible gram-negative cocci, with the exception of staphylococci and, in some cases, enterococci. Penicillin G is the drug of choice for infections caused by certain gram-negative bacilli (eg, *Spirillum minus, Streptobacillus moniliformis, Leptotrichia bucccalis*), actinomycetes, and spirochetes.

Procaine penicillin G and benzathine penicillin G are used to treat infections, such as early syphilis, late latent syphilis, and endocarditis due to penicillin-sensitive streptococci, where prolonged blood levels are needed and frequent dosing of aqueous penicillin G is undesirable. Procaine penicillin G or benzathine penicillin G should not be given when sustained high concentrations of penicillin G are needed. Aqueous penicillin G should be used in this case.

Penicillin V

Penicillin V is more stable than penicillin G in the acid medium of the stomach. As a result, it provides higher blood levels following ingestion. Its absorption is not affected by food. Penicillin V is preferred over penicillin G when oral treatment is indicated.

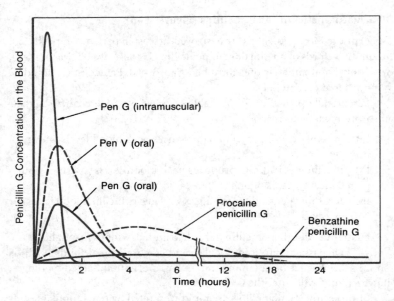

Figure 28–6   Schematic representation of the blood concentration of various forms of penicillin G plotted as a function of time after oral or IM administration. After Pratt WB. Chemotherapy of infections. New York: Oxford Press; 1977.

Narrow-Spectrum, Penicillinase-Resistant Penicillins (Methicillin, Cloxacillin, Dicloxacillin, Flucloxacillin)

Within 5 to 6 years of the introduction of penicillin G and V, most strains of *Staphylococcus aureus* had developed resistance (Figure 28–7) because of their ability to secrete enzymes called penicillinases. Penicillinases are a subgroup of enzymes called beta-lactamases, which rupture the beta-lactam ring of pencillins, thereby inactivating them (Figure 28–8). Bacteria produce a variety of beta-lactamases. Only those beta lactamases that act selectively on penicillin are referred to as penicillinases.

Methicillin, cloxacillin, dicloxacillin, and flucloxacillin are usually resistant to penicillinase secreted by *S. aureus*. Although they are active against many penicillin G–sensitive bacteria, the penicillinase-resistant drugs are not as effective as penicillin G or V against these bacteria. They should be used primarily to treat staphylococcal infections and are considered to have a narrow spectrum of use. Resistant strains of staphylococci have emerged to this entire group of drugs. These bacteria are commonly referred to as methicillin-resistant staphylococci because methicillin was the first drug in this group to be marketed. It is important to understand that the expression "methicillin-resistant staphylococci" means resistance to all penicillinase-resistant

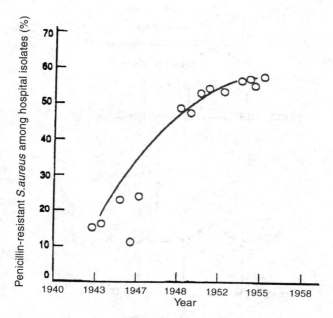

Figure 28–7 Emergence of penicillin-resistant strains of *Staphylococcus aureus* following the widespread introduction of benzylpenicillin (penicillin G) for therapy. (After Richmond MH. Beta-lactam antibiotics, the background to their use as therapeutic agents. Frankfurt: Hoechst Aktiegesellschaft; 1981.)

penicillins. This resistance appears to be due to the production of altered penicillin-binding proteins (PBPs) to which the penicillinase-resistant penicillins are unable to bind. When methicillin-resistant strains of *Staphylococcus aureus* or *S. epidermidis* are known or suspected to be present, vancomycin is the drug of choice.

Expanded-Spectrum Penicillins
1. Aminopenicillins (Ampicillin, Amoxicillin, Bacampicillin, Pivampicillin)

Narrow-spectrum penicillins lack effect against gram-negative bacteria because they cannot cross the outer membrane that surrounds the cell walls of these bacteria. As a result, they cannot reach PBPs on the inner cell membrane to prevent cell wall formation. Aminopenicillins pass through the pores in the outer membrane and reach PBPs on the inner cytoplasmic membrane. These drugs are not resistant to penicillinase secreted by *S. aureus*. They also should not be used to treat penicillin G–sensitive bacteria. The major advantage of the aminopenicillins over penicillin G or V is their activity against most strains of *Escherichia coli, Haemophilus influenzae, Proteus mirabilis, Salmonella,* and *Shigella*.

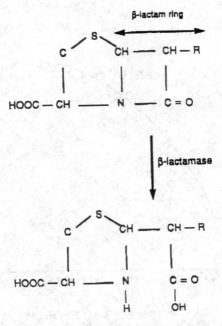

Figure 28–8 Effect of beta-lactamases on the penicillin nucleus. (After Drugs that weaken the bacterial cell wall. 1: Penicillins. In: Lehne RA, Moore LA, Crosby LJ, Hamilton DB, editors. Pharmacology for nursing Care. 2nd ed. Philadelphia: WB Saunders; 1994: pg 929.)

Amoxicillin is preferred over ampicillin for oral administration, because it is more completely absorbed and less likely to cause diarrhea. Bacampicillin and pivampicillin are inactive esters of ampicillin. Once absorbed, they are converted to ampicillin in the body.

2. Antipseudomonal Penicillins (Azlocillin, Mezlocillin, Piperacillin, Ticarcillin)

Antipseudomonal penicillins are effective in higher concentrations against most strains of *Pseudomonas aeruginosa* and indole-negative *Proteus* species. However, their spectrum of activity also covers many other bacteria (see Table 28–2). They are usually used with an aminoglycoside antibiotic, such as gentamicin, tobramycin, amikacin, or netilmicin to treat infections caused by *Pseudomonas* and *Proteus*. The inhibition of cell wall synthesis by the penicillin permits better penetration of the cell wall by the aminoglycoside and more effective inhibition of protein synthesis by the aminoglycoside.

3. Amidino Penicillin (Amdinocillin)

Amdinocillin (mecillinam) is active primarily against gram-negative organisms and relatively ineffective against gram-positive organisms. Amdinocillin pivoxal (pivmecillinam) is a prodrug of amdinocillin that is converted to the microbiologically active amdinocillin (mecillinam) during GI absorption. Pivmecillinam is used to treat acute and chronic urinary tract infections caused by sensitive strains of *E. coli, Klebsiella, Enterobacter,* and *Proteus* species.

4. Penicillins Combined with a Beta-lactamase Inhibitor

By combining a drug that inhibits bacterial beta-lactamases with a penicillinase-sensitive penicillin, it is possible to expand the antimicrobial spectrum of the penicillin. Amoxicillin has been combined with the beta-lactamase inhibitor clavulanic acid. By inhibiting the beta-lactamases secreted by some microorganisms, clavulanic acid protects amoxicillin from hydrolysis and enables it to act against microorganisms that would normally be resistant to the antibiotic. Thus, clavulanic acid increases the spectrum of activity of amoxicillin to include beta-lactamase-producing *Haemophilus influenzae, H. ducreyi, Neisseria gonorrhoeae, Staphylococcus aureus,* and *Branhamella catarrhalis.* Concentrations in the urine will inhibit many strains of *Escherichia coli, Klebsiella, Proteus,* and *Citrobacter.*

Ampicillin has been combined with sulbactam, another beta-lactamase inhibitor. Piperacillin plus tazobactam, and ticarcillin plus clavulanic acid are other combinations of a penicillin plus a beta-lactamase inhibitor. The addition of tazobactam or clavulanic acid to the respective antipseudomonal penicillin extends the spectrum of the penicillin to include staphylococci and a wide variety of anaerobes and gram-negative bacteria.

Adverse Effects

Allergic reactions (Table 28–3) are the major concern with the penicillins. These may occur in 1 to 5% of patients. Patients allergic to one penicillin should be considered allergic to all penicillins.

Given orally, the penicillins may produce GI upset, nausea, vomiting, and diarrhea. Ampicillin is particularly notorious for the burning diarrhea it causes. Amoxicillin is better tolerated.

Table 28–3
Allergic Reactions to Penicillins

Immediate allergic reactions (occur 2–30 minutes after administration)	Urticaria Flushing Diffuse pruritus Hypotension or shock Laryngeal edema Wheezing
Accelerated urticarial reactions (1–71 hours)	Urticaria or pruritus Wheezing or laryngeal edema Local inflammatory reactions
Late allergic reactions (> 72 hours)	Morbilliform eruptions (occasionally occur as early as 18 hours after initiation of treatment) Urticarial eruption Erythematous eruptions Recurrent urticaria and arthralgia Local inflammatory reactions
Some relatively unusual late reactions	Immunohemolytic anemia Drug fever Acute renal insufficiency Thrombocytopenia

THE CEPHALOSPORINS

Antibacterial Spectra

Based on their antibacterial spectra, cephalosporins may be classified as first-, second-, and third-generation (Table 28–4) cephalosporins. They may also be divided into orally and parenterally administered cephalosporins.

Injectable Cephalosporins

First-generation injectable cephalosporins are active against most gram-positive and many gram-negative organisms (Table 28–5).

Second-generation injectable cephalosporins differ little from first-generation drugs with respect to their activity against gram-positive bacteria. They do have, however, lower minimal inhibitory concentrations (MICs) against many gram-negative bacteria. This can be attributed to their:

Table 28–4

Some Currently Available Cephalosporins

First Generation	Second Generation	Third Generation
Cephalothin	Cefamandole	Cefoperazone
Cephapirin	Cefuroxime	Cefotaxime
Cefazolin	Cefoxitin	Ceftazidime
Cephalexin*	Cefaclor*	Ceftizoxime
Cephradine*	Cefonicid	Ceftriaxone
Cefadroxil	Ceforanide	Cefixime*

*Orally active drugs

- increased affinity for the penicillin-binding proteins (PBPs) of gram-negative bacteria,
- increased ability to penetrate the gram-negative cell envelope, and
- increased resistance to beta-lactamases produced by gram-negative organisms.

Third-generation injectable cephalosporins are usually less active than first-generation drugs against staphylococci, but have increased potency and a wider spectrum of activity against clinically important gram-negative bacteria when compared with first- and second-generation cephalosporins. They show excellent activity against many aerobic gram-negative bacilli, including *Haemophilus influenzae* and most of the Enterobacteriaceae, including strains resistant to earlier-generation cephalosporins, penicillins, and aminoglycosides. This activity is due to excellent beta-lactamase stability and their high affinity for PBPs.

Oral Effectiveness

First-generation oral cephalosporins are usually effective against *Staphylococcus aureus,* viridans streptococci, group A streptococci, *Streptococcus pneumoniae, Neisseria meningitidis, N. gonorrhoeae, Salmonella, Shigella, Proteus mirabilis,* and some strains of *Escherichia coli.*

Cefaclor (a second-generation oral cephalosporin) is equivalent to first-generation drugs in activity against gram-positive cocci. It is active against *E. coli, Klebsiella pneumoniae, P. mirabilis, Shigella, Salmonella,* and *H. influenzae.* Cefuroxime axetil is an orally active prodrug of cefuroxime

Table 28–5
Antibacterial Spectrum of Cephalothin, a First-Generation Injectable Cephalosporin

Microorganism	Sensitivity
Staphylococcus aureus (both penicillin sensitive and penicillin resistant)	High sensitivity, but some resistant strains
Streptococcus pyogenes	High sensitivity
Streptococcus pneumoniae	High sensitivity
Streptococcus (viridans group)	High sensitivity
Streptococcus faecalis	Some sensitivity, but many resistant strains
Clostridium perfringens	High sensitivity
Clostridium tetani	Very high sensitivity
Corynebacterium diphtheriae	Some sensitivity
Enterobacter cloacae	Resistant
Enterobacter aerogenes	Resistant
Escherichia coli	Moderate sensitivity, but many resistant strains
Haemophilus influenzae	Moderate sensitivity, but many resistant strains
Klebsiella pneumoniae	High sensitivity
Neisseria gonorrhoeae	Moderate sensitivity, but many resistant strains
Neisseria meningitidis	High sensitivity, but many resistant strains
Proteus mirabilis	Some sensitivity
Proteus morganii	Resistant
Proteus rettgeri	Resistant
Proteus vulgaris	Resistant
Pseudomonas aeruginosa	Resistant
Salmonella spp.	Moderate sensitivity, but many resistant strains
Shigella spp.	Moderate sensitivity, but many resistant strains

that is hydrolyzed by nonspecific esterases to release cefuroxime into the blood stream.

Cefixime (a third-generation oral cephalosporin) is at least as active as other oral cephalosporins against group A streptococci and pneumococci, but staphylococci, which are susceptible to other cephalosporins, are resistant to cefixime because the drug has a low affinity for a critical PBP. Cefixime is highly active against *Neisseria gonorrhoeae, Haemophilus influenzae,* and *Moraxella catarrhalis,* including beta-lactamase-producing strains usually resistant to ampicillin, amoxicillin, and occasionally to cefaclor. Cefixime is more active than other cephalosporins against many gram-negative bacilli, including *E. coli, Klebsiella, Proteus mirabilis,* and *Serratia marcescens.*

Resistance

Resistance can develop to cephalosporins by several means, including:

1. inactivation by bacteria beta-lactamases,
2. decreased permeability of the bacterial cells, which prevents the cephalosporin from reaching the appropriate binding proteins, and
3. alterations in the penicillin-binding proteins that prevent the cephalosporins from binding to them.

Clinically, beta-lactamase inactivation and, to a lesser extent, altered permeability are most important in gram-negative bacteria. The rapid development of resistance to supposedly beta-lactamase-stable third-generation cephalosporins, particularly by species of *Enterobacter, Serratia,* and *Pseudomonas,* is of increasing concern.

Adverse Effects

Cephalosporins are relatively safe drugs, but they can produce allergic reactions in as many as 5% of patients. These include skin rash, urticaria, fever, serum sickness, hemolytic anemia, and eosinophilia.

GI adverse effects include nausea, vomiting, and diarrhea. Overgrowth of resistant organisms may occur after long-term cephalosporin administration. Patients receiving a third-generation cephalosporin should be observed for enterococcal superinfection. Finally, third-generation cephalosporins may suppress the GI microflora, resulting in decreased vitamin K production and hypoprothrombinemia.

29

Macrolide Antibiotics

ERYTHROMYCIN, CLARITHROMYCIN, AZITHROMYCIN

Actions

Macrolide antibiotics inhibit bacterial protein synthesis by reversibly binding to the 50S ribosomal subunit and preventing elongation of the peptide chain, most likely by interfering with the translocation step. Macrolides do not bind to mammalian 50S ribosomes, and this partly accounts for their selective toxicity.

Macrolides may be bacteriostatic or bactericidal, depending on the concentration of the drug, organism susceptibility, growth rate, and size of the inoculum. Bacterial killing is favored by higher antibiotic concentrations, lower bacterial density, and rapid growth.

Antibacterial Spectra

Erythromycin

Erythromycin has an antibacterial spectrum similar to that of penicillin G. It includes many strains of penicillin-resistant staphylococci, *Streptococcus pyogenes, Streptococcus pneumoniae,* viridans streptococci, anaerobic streptococci, and many strains of *Streptococcus faecalis.* Erythromycin is also effective against *Corynebacterium diphtheriae, Propionibacterium acnes, Clostridium tetani, Clostridium perfringens, Neisseria gonorrhoeae, Bordetella pertussis,* and some species of *Brucella. Haemophilus influenzae* is only moderately sensitive to the drug. Oropharyngeal strains of *Bacteroides* are usually sensitive to erythromycin. The drug is also effective against *Mycoplasma pneumoniae, Treponema pallidum, Legionella pneumophila,* and many species of *Rickettsia* and *Chlamydia.*

Clarithromycin

Clarithromycin has an in vitro spectrum of activity that is similar to that of erythromycin, but it is two- to fourfold more active against susceptible streptococci and staphylococci. Gram-positive cocci resistant to erythromycin are resistant to clarithromycin as well. Clarithromycin is slightly more active in vitro than erythromycin against certain pathogens responsible for atypical pneumonias (ie, *Legionella pneumophila, Mycoplasma pneumoniae, Chlamydia pneumoniae*).

Azithromycin

Azithromycin, unlike erythromycin and clarithromycin, inhibits some aerobic gram-negative bacilli. The majority of these bacilli, including the Enterobacteriaceae, are intrinsically resistant to erythromycin and clarithromycin because the cell envelopes prevent passive diffusion of the antibiotic. Organisms that are moderately susceptible to azithromycin include most *Salmonella, Shigella* and *Aeromonas* species, *Escherichia coli,* and *Yersinia enterocolitica.* Azithromycin has excellent activity against *Vibrio cholerea* and species isolated in patients with vaginitis, such as *Gardnerella vaginalis* and *Mobiluncus.*

Resistance

Bacteria with developed resistance to erythromycin are also resistant to azithromycin and clarithromycin. Plasmid-mediated decreased binding of macrolides to their target site accounts for nearly all the resistant strains isolated from patients.

Pharmacokinetics

Erythromycin

Erythromycin is not stable in the stomach; it must be protected from gastric juices. This can be achieved by using enteric-coated tablets or capsules, or by preparing the drug as an acid-resistant ester, such as erythromycin stearate, erythromycin ethylsuccinate, or erythromycin estolate, which are hydrolyzed to erythromycin once absorbed. Once absorbed, erythromycin diffuses well throughout the body. It enters most tissue compartments, with the exception of the CSF. Erythromycin is concentrated in the liver and excreted in the bile. Little erythromycin is eliminated in urine. Its half-life ranges from 1 to more than 3 hours.

Clarithromycin

Clarithromycin is well absorbed from the GI tract, with or without food. It is metabolized in the liver, and 30 to 40% of the administered dose can be recovered in the urine. Patients with a creatinine clearance ≤ 30 mL/min may require a decreased dose. Clarithromycin penetrates well into both tissues and cells, including macrophages and polymorphonuclear leukocytes. Clarithromycin is 65 to 70% bound to plasma proteins.

Azithromycin

Azithromycin is rapidly absorbed and distributed widely throughout the body. Rapid movement of azithromycin from blood into tissue results in significantly higher azithromycin concentrations in tissue than in plasma (up to 50 times the maximum observed concentration in plasma). The absolute bioavailability is approximately 37%. Following its absorption, azithromycin is eliminated slowly from the body. Its half-life is 68 hours. Elimination in the bile, metabolism in the liver, and possibly transintestinal elimination account for the clearance of azithromycin from the body.

Uses

Erythromycin

Erythromycin is often used as a replacement for penicillin G or V in patients who are allergic to these drugs. It can be used in the following ways:

1. In the treatment of infections caused by group A streptococci, including tonsillitis, erysipelas, and scarlet fever
2. As a penicillin substitute in the chemoprophylaxis of streptococcal infections
3. To treat pneumococcal infections
4. As a substitute for penicillin in the treatment of the acute illness or carrier state of diphtheria and in the management of both early and late syphilis
5. In the treatment of *Mycoplasma pneumoniae* and Legionnaire's disease caused by *Legionella pneumophila*
6. To treat *Chylamydia trachomatis* infections in infants and children
7. In conjunction with sulfisoxazole to treat *Haemophilus influenzae*–induced otitis media in young children
8. In the treatment of acne vulgaris

Erythromycin can eradicate *Propionibacterium acnes*, the anaerobic diphtheroid in pilosebaceous glands that secretes a variety of enzymes, including hyaluronidase, which are capable of disrupting follicular epithelium and increasing inflammation.

Clarithromycin

Clarithromycin is used to treat:

1. Pneumonia caused by *Mycoplasma pneumoniae* or *Streptococcus pneumoniae*
2. Acute bacterial exacerbations of chronic bronchitis due to *H. influenzae, Moraxella catarrhalis,* or *S. pneumoniae*
3. Pharyngitis/tonsillitis due to *Streptococcus pyogenes*
4. Acute maxillary sinusitis due to *S. pneumoniae* in penicillin-allergic patients
5. Uncomplicated skin and skin-structure infections due to *S. aureus* or *S. pyogenes*

Azithromycin

Azithromycin is used in the following ways:

1. As an alternative antibiotic for the treatment of mild to moderate pharyngitis/tonsillitis due to streptococcal species
2. To treat mild to moderate acute bacterial exacerbations of chronic bronchitis due to *H. influenzae, M. catarrhalis,* or *S. pneumoniae*
3. In the treatment of pneumonia due to *S. pneumoniae* or *H. influenzae*
4. To treat uncomplicated skin and skin-structure infections due to *S. aureus, S. pyogenes* or *Streptococcus agalactiae*
5. In the treatment of urethritis and cervicitis due to *C. trachomatis*

Adverse Effects

Erythromycin is well tolerated, except for its effects on the GI tract. Erythromycin causes GI upset with nausea, diarrhea, and abdominal pain.

Both **clarithromycin and azithromycin** are well tolerated. Neither drug causes the high incidence of disabling nausea seen with erythromycin. Reversible dose-related hearing loss has been reported with high doses (eg, ≥ 4 g/24 h) of both drugs used to treat *Mycobacterium avium* infections.

30

Aminoglycoside Antibiotics

AMIKACIN, GENTAMICIN, NETILMICIN, TOBRAMYCIN

Actions

Aminoglycoside antibiotics are a group of structurally related bactericidal drugs. They derive their name from the fact that their structures contain at least one sugar attached to one or more amino groups. Aminoglycosides inhibit bacterial protein synthesis. They bind to the 30S ribosomal subunit of streptococci to cause a misreading of the genetic code. The proteins formed contain the wrong sequence of amino acids and have no biologic value ("nonsense proteins"). Aminoglycosides block protein synthesis in other bacteria by inhibiting amino acid translocation.

Antibacterial Spectrum

Aminoglycosides are principally used to treat infections caused by sensitive strains of Enterobacteriaceae, including *Escherichia coli, Klebsiella, Enterobacter, Serratia*, and *Proteus* species. Amikacin, gentamicin, netilmicin, and tobramycin are active against *Pseudomonas aeruginosa*. They have only limited activity against most gram-positive bacteria. They are active in vitro against certain species of streptococcus. Only minimal activity is usually found against *Streptococcus faecalis, S. pneumoniae,* and streptococci of the viridans group. Although aminoglycosides inhibit staphylococci, safer drugs such as the penicillins or cephalosporins, are usually used against these pathogens. Aminoglycosides have little activity against anaerobic microorganisms or facultative bacteria under anaerobic conditions.

Although the antibacterial spectra of amikacin, gentamicin, netilmicin, and tobramycin show few qualitative differences, the various aerobic gram-

252

negative bacilli vary in their susceptibility to the four drugs. Table 30–1 describes the differing sensitivities of six gram-negative bacilli to tobramycin and gentamicin.

Resistance

Bacterial resistance can develop to the aminoglycosides. The major mechanism for the development of resistance involves enzymatic inactivation of the antibiotics. Decreased uptake of the aminoglycoside by bacteria or alteration of bacterial ribosomal binding sites can also account for the development of resistance.

The aminoglycosides are inactivated by acetylation, adenylation, or phosphorylation of critical binding sites. The prevalence of individual aminoglycoside inactivating enzymes varies widely, both with respect to geographic location and time. Thus, different patterns of aminoglycoside resistance exist among countries, among hospitals in any country, district, or city, and even among wards within a hospital. Therefore, established tests of sensitivity should be used to determine bacterial susceptibility to a drug.

Pharmacokinetics

The aminoglycosides are very polar (water-soluble) drugs and cannot diffuse across gastrointestinal membranes. Less than 1% of an oral dose is absorbed. Aminoglycosides are absorbed rapidly from IM injection sites, with peak concentrations appearing within 1 hour.

Aminoglycosides do not diffuse readily across body membranes. For example, concentrations of gentamicin in pleural and pericardial fluids are

Table 30–1
In Vitro Activity of Tobramycin and Gentamicin Against Susceptible Gram-Negative Organisms

	Number of Strains	Tobramycin (%)*	Gentamicin (%)*
Escherichia coli	100	93	80
Enterobacter spp.	52	94	81
Proteus mirabilis	38	92	58
Proteus spp. (indole positive)	26	100	85
Klebsiella spp.	100	100	98
Serratia marcescens	41	86	88

*Percentage of isolates susceptible to 1.57 µg/mL.

only one-quarter to one-half those in serum. Aminoglycoside levels in fetal serum are 20 to 40% of those in maternal serum. Aminoglycosides do not cross well into the CSF, even in the presence of inflammation.

Aminoglycosides are eliminated by renal excretion. Their half-lives of 2 to 3 hours in patients with normal kidney function are extended in patients with renal impairment. Dosages must be decreased in the neonate or adult with reduced renal function.

Uses

Gentamicin is still important in the treatment of many serious gram-negative bacillary infections (eg, caused by *E. coli, Proteus mirabilis,* indole-positive *Proteus, Klebsiella, Enterobacter*, and *Serratia* species and *Pseudomonas aeruginosa*), although resistance to the drug is developing. *Salmonella* and *Shigella* species are often gentamicin-sensitive.

Gentamicin can be considered for the treatment of bacteremia, respiratory and urinary tract infections, infected wounds, and bone and soft-tissue infections, including peritonitis and burns complicated by sepsis. Serious infections with *P. aeruginosa* may require gentamicin combined with carbenicillin, ticarcillin, pipracillin, or ceftazidime. The combination produces a synergistic effect with some strains and delays the emergence of resistant organisms.

Gentamicin is also applied topically for use in the treatment of primary and secondary infections caused by sensitive strains of streptococcus (Group A beta-hemolytic, alpha-hemolytic), *Staphylococcus aureus* (coagulase-positive, coagulase-negative, and some penicillinase-producing strains), and the gram-negative bacteria *P. aeruginosa, Aerobacter aerogenes, E. coli, Proteus vulgaris,* and *Klebsiella pneumoniae.* Gentamicin may also be used for ocular infections caused by *S. aureus, P. aeruginosa, A. aerogenes, E. coli, Proteus vulgaris,* or *K. pneumoniae.*

Tobramycin has a similar antibacterial spectrum to that of gentamicin. It is usually active against most strains of the following organisms in vitro and in clinical infections: *P. aeruginosa; Proteus* species (indole positive and indole-negative), including *P. mirabilis, P. morganii, P. rettgeri,* and *P. vulgaris; E. coli; Klebsiella-Enterobacter-Serratia* group; *Citrobacter* species; *Providencia* species; and staphylococci, including *S. aureus* (coagulase positive and coagulase negative). Its minimum inhibitory concentration (MIC) against *P. aeruginosa* is approximately one-quarter that of gentamicin. Tobramycin is considered by many to be the aminoglycoside of choice for *P. aeruginosa* infections, in which case it is combined with carbenicillin, ticarcillin, piperacillin, or ceftazidime.

Tobramycin may be indicated for the treatment of the following infections when caused by susceptible organisms: septicemia, urinary tract infections, lower respiratory tract infections, serious skin and soft-tissue infections, and CNS infections resistant to antibiotics usually considered efficacious in such infections.

Like gentamicin, tobramycin can be used topically for ocular infections caused by *S. aureus, P. aeruginosa, A. aerogenes, E. coli, P. vulgaris,* or *K. pneumoniae.*

Amikacin is indicated for the short-term treatment of serious infections due to amikacin-susceptible strains of *P. aeruginosa, E. coli,* and *S. aureus,* as well as *Proteus, Klebsiella-Enterobacter-Serratia, Providencia, Salmonella,* and *Citrobacter* species. Among the aminoglycosides, amikacin has the greatest resistance to bacterial aminoglycoside-inactivating enzymes. Amikacin is often considered to be the drug of choice for the initial treatment of serious gram-negative bacillary infections in hospitals, where gentamicin resistance is a problem.

Netilmicin has a similar spectrum of activity to that of gentamicin and tobramycin. However, because it is less sensitive to bacterial inactivation, netilmicin is effective against some gentamicin-resistant and tobramycin-resistant strains of Enterobacteriaceae. Netilmicin is indicated for the treatment of infections caused by susceptible strains of *E. coli, Proteus* (indole negative and some indole positive), *Klebsiella, Enterobacter, Citrobacter,* and *Staphylococcus* species.

Adverse Effects

Aminoglycosides accumulate in the perilymph of the inner ear, destroying both the vestibular and cochlear sensory cells. The degree of permanent damage correlates with the number of destroyed sensory hair cells in the inner ear; this in turn relates to the concentration of the drug and length of exposure. Patients experience tinnitus and hearing loss, dizziness, and vertigo. Amikacin impairs auditory function preferentially, and gentamicin is more likely to damage vestibular function. Tobramycin causes auditory and vestibular damage with equal frequency. The diuretics ethacrynic acid and furosemide potentiate aminoglycoside ototoxicity.

High concentrations of aminoglycosides accumulate in the renal cortex and urine. Five to 7 days of therapy can cause dose-dependent damage in the proximal tubular epithelium, particularly in elderly or debilitated patients or in individuals with pre-existing renal impairment. Serum creatinine and blood urea nitrogen increase, and severe azotemia may occur. Tobramycin and netilmicin are claimed to be less nephrotoxic than the other aminoglycosides. Concomitant therapy with furosemide, ethacrynic acid, cephalosporins, or methoxyflurane increases the risk of the nephrotoxicity.

Rarely, aminoglycosides can reduce the release of acetylcholine from motor nerve terminals and cause a neuromuscular blockade, leading to a flaccid paralysis and respiratory failure.

31

Fluoroquinolone Antibiotics

CIPROFLOXACIN, ENOXACIN, LOMEFLOXACIN, NORFLOXACIN, OFLOXACIN

Actions

Fluoroquinolones (Figure 31–1) inhibit DNA synthesis by a specific action on DNA gyrase, the enzyme responsible for the unwinding and supercoiling of bacterial DNA within the bacterium before its replication.

Antibacterial Spectrum

Fluoroquinolones are effective against most aerobic, gram-negative, and some gram-positive bacteria. The fluoroquinolones are highly active against Enterobacteriaceae, including *Escherichia coli, Klebsiella, Enterobacter, Proteus mirabilis, Proteus vulgaris, Morganella morganii, Providencia, Citrobacter,* and *Serratia.* These drugs are active against *Pseudomonas aeruginosa,* including strains that are resistant to other antibacterials.

The gram-negative coccobacilli *Haemophilus influenzae* and *Haemophilus ducreyi,* and the gram-negative cocci *Neisseria meningitidis, Neisseria gonorrhoeae,* and *Moraxella catarrhalis,* are highly susceptible to the fluoroquinolones. The beta-lactamase–producing strains of these organisms are also susceptible.

The fluoroquinolones are active against some gram-positive bacteria, although inhibitory concentrations generally are higher than for gram-negative bacteria. All of the fluoroquinolones are active against staphylococci (*Staphylococcus aureus, Staphylococcus epidermidis*), including methicillin-resistant strains.

Streptococci, including *Streptococcus pyogenes* (group A), *Streptococcus agaletiae* (group B), *Streptococcus pneumoniae,* and viridans streptococci, are usually highly susceptible.

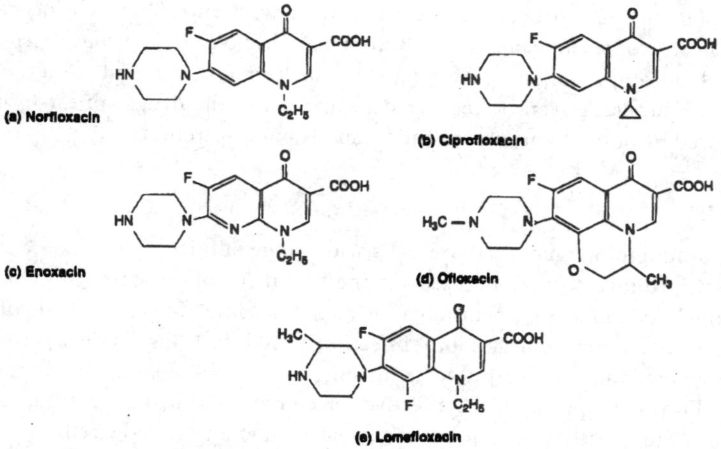

Figure 31–1 Chemical structures of fluoroquinolones. After AMA Drug Evaluations Subscriptions; 1993, 2:13. p. 8:2.

The fluoroquinolones are active in vitro against *Legionella pneumophila*. Ciprofloxacin and ofloxacin are active against *Mycobacterium tuberculosis* and certain atypical mycobacteria.

Resistance

Plasmid-mediated transferable resistance to the fluoroquinolones has been reported. However, resistance can be caused by chromosomal mutations. These involve alterations in DNA gyrase or changes in outer membrane proteins that affect bacterial membrane permeability.

Pharmacokinetics

The fluoroquinolones are rapidly, but variably absorbed following oral administration. Oral bioavailability is approximately 40 to 50% for norfloxacin, 60 to 70% for ciprofloxacin, and 90 to 100% for enoxacin, lomefloxacin, and ofloxacin.

All the fluoroquinolones appear to distribute widely in body fluids and tissues. They penetrate into blister fluid, bile, saliva, sputum, peritoneal fluid, macrophages, polymorphonuclear neutrophils, lung, liver, kidney, gall bladder, skeletal muscle, uterus, cervix, vagina, and bone. In the urine, all the fluoroquinolones reach concentrations that exceed the MIC of most urinary tract pathogens for at least 12 hours.

In patients with inflamed meninges, ciprofloxacin and ofloxacin may reach concentrations in the CSF that exceed the MIC90 for most gram-negative pathogens that cause bacterial meningitis, including *Pseudomonas aeruginosa, Salmonella* species, and other Enterobacteriaceae. However, the CSF levels of these drugs are not adequate to treat meningitis caused by staphylococci, *Streptococcus pneumoniae*, group B streptococci, and *Listeria monocytogenes*.

Fluoroquinolones are eliminated by the liver, GI tract, and kidney. All fluoroquinolones can be recovered in urine, and the drugs appear to be cleared by both glomerular filtration and tubular secretion.

Uses

Fluoroquinolones are used to treat a wide range of infections.

Ciprofloxacin may be used for the treatment of patients with acute bronchitis and acute pneumonia, urinary tract infections, skin and soft-tissue infections, bone and joint infections, and infectious diarrhea caused by a wide range of susceptible organisms.

Enoxacin appears to be effective for complicated urinary tract infections. Single doses have been beneficial in uncomplicated urethral and endocervical gonorrhea.

Lomefloxacin is used in acute exacerbations of chronic bronchitis of mixed etiology that does not involve *S. pneumoniae*. It is also used in uncomplicated and complicated infections of the upper and lower urinary tract. Lomefloxacin appears to be effective in the treatment of acute and chronic bacterial prostatitis, infectious diarrhea, bone and joint infections, infections of the skin and skin structures, and sexually transmitted diseases (eg, chancroid due to *H. ducreyi*).

Norfloxacin is indicated for the treatment of upper and lower urinary tract infections (specifically complicated and uncomplicated cystitis), pyelitis, and pyelonephritis caused by susceptible strains of *E. coli, Klebsiella pneumoniae*, unspecified *Klebsiella*, unspecified *Citrobacter, P. mirabilis, S. aureus, Streptococcus faecalis*, and *P. aeruginosa*.

Ofloxacin is used to treat lower respiratory tract infections, including pneumonia, and acute exacerbations of chronic bronchitis due to *H. influenzae or S. pneumoniae*. It is also used to treat uncomplicated cystitis or complicated urinary tract infections due to *E. coli, K. pneumoniae*, or *P. mirabilis*. Ofloxacin is used to treat prostatitis due to *E. coli*. Sexually transmitted disease due to *N. gonorrhoeae* and nongonococcal urethritis and cervicitis due to *Chlamydia trachomatis* can also be treated with ofloxacin. Finally, ofloxacin can be used in mild to moderate skin and skin-structure infections due to *S. aureus* and *S. pyogenes*.

Adverse Effects

The fluoroquinolones are well tolerated and rarely require discontinuation because of adverse effects. Nausea, vomiting, and dizziness occur most commonly. Abdominal pain, dyspepsia, flatulence, vomiting, diarrhea, and stomatitis are also encountered. CNS adverse effects include malaise, drowsiness, weakness, insomnia, restlessness, and agitation.

32

Miscellaneous Antibiotics and Antibacterials

COTRIMOXAZOLE (TRIMETHOPRIM PLUS SULFAMETHOXAZOLE

Actions

Cotrimoxazole contains sulfamethoxazole plus trimethoprim.

- **Sulfamethoxazole (SMZ)** is a sulfonamide drug, which inhibits bacterial folic acid synthesis. Humans absorb folic acid from food, but bacteria must synthesize the vitamin. Para-aminobenzoic acid (PABA) is an essential component of folic acid. Sulfonamides, like SMZ (Figure 32–1), are structurally similar to PABA. By acting as competitive antimetabolites of PABA, sulfonamides block PABA's incorporation into folic acid (Figure 32–2), thereby preventing folic acid synthesis and inducing bacteriostasis. Because humans can absorb folic acid from food and bacteria must synthesize the vitamin, sulfonamides are selectively toxic to bacteria.
- **Trimethoprim (TMP)** (see Figure 32–1) competitively inhibits bacterial dihydrofolate reductase, the enzyme responsible for converting dihydrofolic acid to tetrahydrofolic acid, the active form of folic acid.
- **Cotrimoxazole** is an effective combination, in which SMZ reduces folic acid synthesis and TMP inhibits folic acid activation (Figure 32–3).

Antibacterial Spectrum

Cotrimoxazole has a broad spectrum of activity. All strains of *Staphylococcus aureus, Streptococcus pneumoniae, Streptococcus epidermidis, Streptococ-*

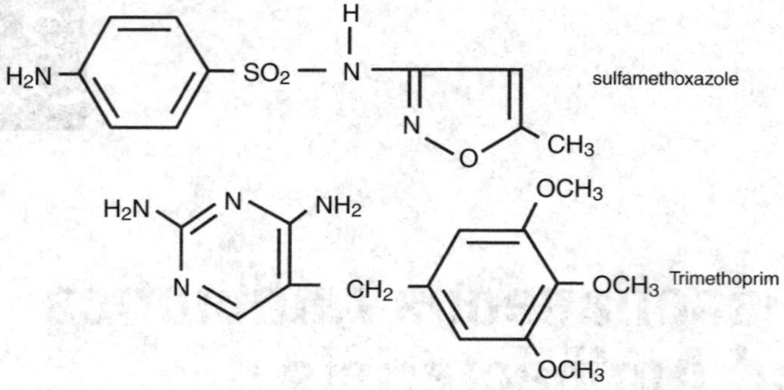

Figure 32-1 Structures of sulfamethoxazole and trimethoprim.

cus pyogenes, viridans streptococci, *Streptococcus faecalis*, *Escherichia coli*, *Proteus mirabilis*, *Proteus morganii*, *Proteus rettgeri*, *Enterobacter* species, *Pseudomonas psueudomallei*, and *Serratia* species are inhibited by cotrimoxazole. Although many strains of *Shigella* and *Salmonella* remain sensitive to cotrimoxazole, others have developed resistance to it.

Resistance

Resistance can develop to cotrimoxazole. This may be either plasmid- or chromosome-mediated. Clinically, the most important type of acquired

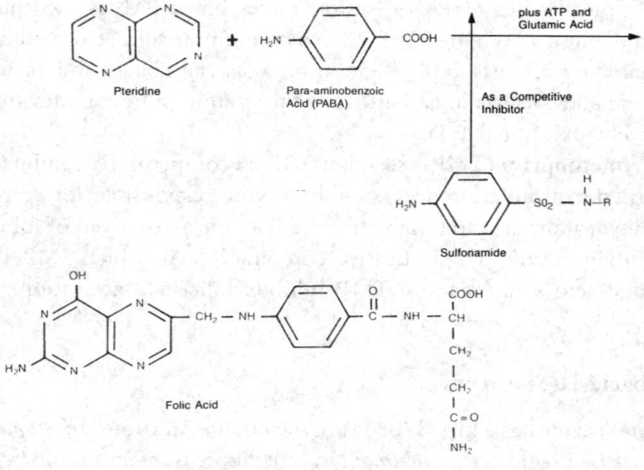

Figure 32-2 Mechanism of action of sulfonamides.

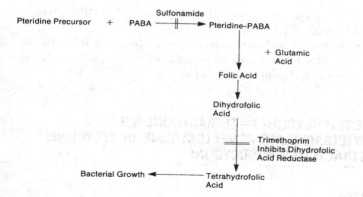

Figure 32–3 Mechanism of action of cotrimoxazole.

resistance to TMP results from the production of novel TMP-resistant dihydrofolate reductase. These dihydrofolate reductase enzymes are encoded on transferable plasmids or transposons and confer on the bacteria a high-level of resistance to TMP.

Pharmacokinetics

Both SMZ and TMP are well absorbed from the GI tract and distribute rapidly throughout the body, including the CSF. High concentrations of each drug are found in the bile. The half-life of both drugs is approximately 10 hours. Although most of the TMP is eliminated unchanged in the urine, approximately 85% of SMZ is inactivated prior to renal excretion.

Uses

Cotrimoxazole is used to treat a variety of systemic infections caused by gram-positive and gram-negative organisms, including infections of the upper and lower respiratory tract, urinary tract, genitourinary tract, gastrointestinal tract, and skin and soft tissues; *Pneumocystis carinii* infections; and serious systemic infections, such as meningitis and septicemia caused by susceptible organisms.

Adverse Effects

Nausea, anorexia, and vomiting are seen in 5 to 10% of patients taking sulfonamides. Hypersensitivity reactions to sulfonamides, beginning 10 to 12 days after starting therapy or within hours in previously sensitized patients, can cause generalized skin rashes, urticaria, photodermatitis, or drug fever. Blood dyscrasias to sulfonamides are rare but they can be fatal. Acute or chronic hemolytic anemia, developing within 2 to 7 days of starting sulfonamide therapy, or agranulocytosis, appearing between the second and sixth week of treatment, represent hypersensitivity reactions.

TMP has relatively few adverse effects. They include gastric distress (nausea and vomiting), rash, itching, and very rarely, leukopenia, thrombocytopenia, and methemoglobinemia.

THE TETRACYCLINES—TETRACYCLINE HCl, OXYTETRACYCLINE, DEMECLOCYCLINE, DOXYCYCLINE, METHACYCLINE, MINOCYCLINE

Actions

All tetracyclines have the same basic structure (Figure 32–4) and the same bacteriostatic mechanism of action. Tetracyclines are concentrated within sensitive gram-positive and gram-negative bacterial cells by an energy-dependent process. Once inside the bacteria, tetracyclines depress protein synthesis by blocking the attachment of aminoacyl transfer RNA to the acceptor site on the messenger RNA-ribosome complex. Binding of the tetracycline antibiotic occurs primarily at the bacterial 30S ribosomal subunit.

The selective toxicity of tetracyclines for sensitive bacteria, and their safety to the host, appears to depend partially on the energy-dependent uptake of the antibiotics by bacterial, and not mammalian, cells.

Antibacterial Spectrum

Table 32–1 presents the antibacterial spectrum of the tetracyclines.

Resistance

Several species of bacteria have become increasingly resistant to the tetracyclines. Many enterobacteriaceae (eg, *Shigella, Escherichia coli*) and most *Pseudomonas aeruginosa* are resistant. Many strains of staphylococci, streptococci, pneumococci, and *Bacteroides* are no longer susceptible. Emergence of high-level tetracycline-resistant *Neisseria gonorrhoeae* strains is common in some areas of the world.

Pharmacokinetics

Absorption from the GI tract ranges from 60 to 80% for oxytetracycline, tetracycline, and demeclocycline and from 95 to 100% for minocycline and doxycycline. Calcium, magnesium, and iron block tetracycline absorption.

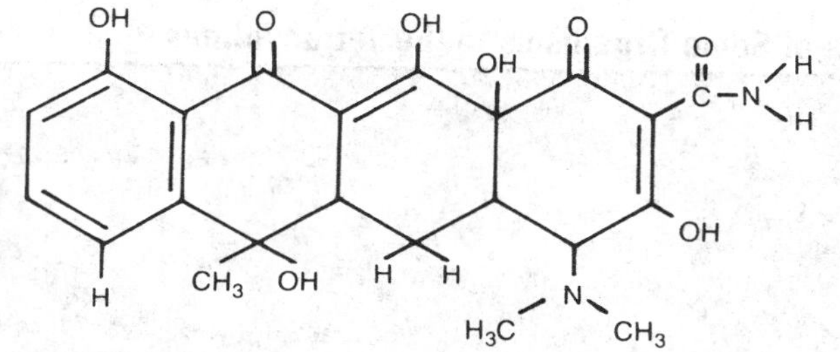

Tetracycline

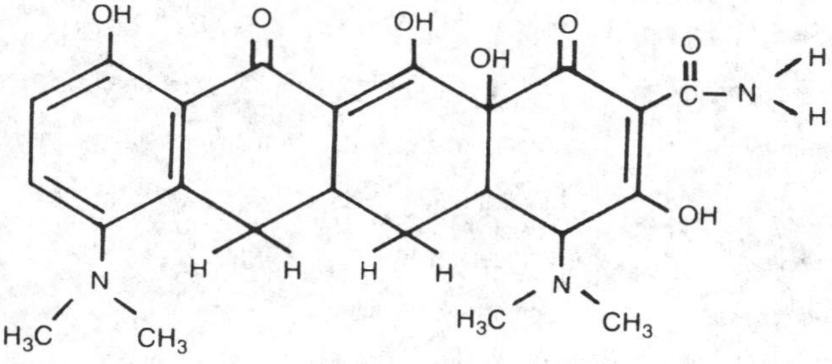

Minocycline

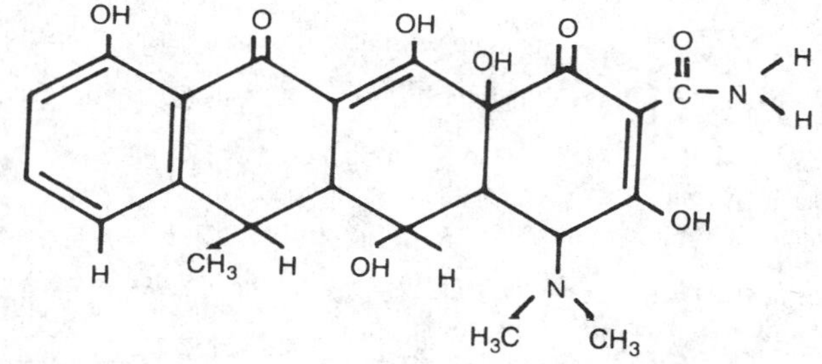

Doxycycline

Figure 32–4 Structure of tetracycline, minocycline, and doxycycline.

Distribution in the body differs among the tetracyclines. Oxytetracycline, tetracycline, and minocycline are 35, 65, and 75% bound to the plasma proteins, respectively. Methacycline, demeclocycline, and doxycycline are approximately 90% bound to plasma albumin. Tetracyclines distribute to varying degrees throughout the body. They cross the placenta but have difficulty crossing the blood-brain barrier. Doxycycline and minocycline are more lipophilic and penetrate tissues and secretions better than the other tetracyclines. Doxycycline diffuses well into endometrial, myometrial, prostatic, and renal tissues.

Tetracyclines bind to calcium and are retained in bone and growing teeth for long periods of time. Because they can damage developing teeth and delay the development of long bones, tetracyclines are usually contraindicated during pregnancy and in patients under 8 to 10 years of age.

Table 32–1
Sensitivities of Some Organisms to the Tetracyclines

Bacillus anthracis	Some sensitivity
Bacteroides spp.	Moderate sensitivity, but many resistant strains
Clostridium perfringens	Moderate sensitivity
Clostridium tetani	Moderate sensitivity
Escherichia coli	Moderate sensitivity, but many resistant strains
Haemophilus ducreyi	High sensitivity, but many resistant strains
Haemophilus influenzae	High sensitivity, but many resistant strains
Klebsiella pneumoniae	Moderate sensitivity, but many resistant strains
Listeria monocytogenes	Moderate sensitivity
Mycoplasma pneumoniae	High sensitivity
Neisseria gonorrhoeae	Moderate sensitivity
Neisseria meningitidis	Moderate sensitivity
Salmonella spp.	Moderate sensitivity, but many resistant strains
Shigella spp.	Moderate sensitivity, but many resistant strains
Staphylococcus aureus (both penicillin sensitive and penicillin resistant)	Some sensitivity, but tetracyclines not recommended for treatment
Streptococcus pneumoniae	Moderate sensitivity, but some areas have many resistant strains
Streptococcus pyogenes	Moderate sensitivity, but many resistant strains
Treponema pallidum	Sensitive; tetracycline is recommended in penicillin-allergic patients

Elimination rates differ among the tetracyclines. The half-lives range from 8 to 9 hours (for tetracycline HCl and oxytetracycline) to 16 to 18 hours (for minocycline and doxycycline). Renal excretion is the major route of elimination. Minocycline has a low renal clearance, and less than 10% of a dose is recovered unchanged in urine. The drug undergoes entero-hepatic circulation and may be metabolized to a considerable extent. Doxy-cycline elimination is independent of both renal and hepatic function. The drug is excreted in the feces, largely as an inactive chelated product. Thus, the dose of doxycycline does not require modification in patients with renal or hepatic insufficiency.

Uses

Despite their broad antibacterial spectrum, tetracyclines have relatively poor activity against most pathogens and are rarely considered drugs of first choice. They are considered first-line drugs for the treatment of *Mycoplasma pneumoniae,* Rocky Mountain spotted fever, endemic typhus, *Borrelia recurrentis* (relapsing fever), chlamydial disease, nonspecific brucellosis, and infections caused by *Pasteurella.* For most infections, tetracyclines are second- or third-line drugs, falling behind more effective agents.

Minocycline is frequently prescribed for the treatment of acne vulgaris. By eradicating the anaerobe *Propionibacterium acnes,* minocycline reduces the production of inflammatory fatty acids by the microbe and decreases inflammatory acne. Minocycline is also used to treat rosacea. Exactly why minocycline should be effective in rosacea is not known. However, its efficacy is probably unrelated to its antibacterial properties.

Adverse Effects

Tetracyclines can cause nausea, vomiting, epigastric burning, stomatitis, and glossitis when given orally. Administered intravenously, they can produce phlebitis. Tetracyclines can be hepatotoxic, particularly in patients with pre-existing renal or hepatic insufficiency.

Tetracyclines can retard bone growth in the developing fetus if given to pregnant women after the fourth month of gestation. They can also stain teeth and retard growth if given to children under 8 years.

Photosensitivity, manifested mainly as abnormal sunburn reactions, is particularly prevalent with demeclocycline. Minocycline produces vertigo in a high percentage of patients.

Tetracyclines can produce superinfections. By suppressing the normal bacterial flora, tetracyclines enable other bacteria, such as penicillinase-producing staphylococci and *Candida,* to proliferate. Superinfections occur in the oral, anogenital, and intestinal areas.

Tetracyclines can also lead to pseudomembranous colitis, secondary to the overgrowth of *Clostridium difficile.*

VANCOMYCIN

Actions

Vancomycin inhibits cell wall synthesis in susceptible bacteria. However, it is structurally and pharmacodynamically very different from beta-lactam antibiotics, which also inhibit cell wall synthesis. Vancomycin does not bind to penicillin-binding proteins (PBPs) (see Chapter 28), but instead binds to a different component of the cell wall to interfere with the elongation of the peptidoglycan backbone of the wall. This specificity of action partly explains the minimal resistance shown to vancomycin to date.

Antibacterial Spectrum

Vancomycin is only active against gram-positive bacteria. Because it cannot penetrate the outer membrane that surrounds gram-negative species, vancomycin is ineffective in treating gram-negative infections. Vancomycin is one of the most potent antibiotics against *Staphylococcus aureus* and *S. epidermidis*, including methicillin- and cephalothin-resistant strains (Chapter 28).

Streptococcus pyogenes and *S. pneumoniae* (including penicillin G–resistant strains) are highly susceptible to vancomycin. The drug usually inhibits the growth of viridans streptococcus, *Streptococcus bovis, Streptococcus agalactiae* (group B), and enterococci (*eg, Enterobacter faecalis*). However, vancomycin may not be bactericidal against some strains of these species, particularly the enterococci. Antibacterial synergism against enterococci is usually obtained when vancomycin is combined with an aminoglycoside.

Gram-positive bacilli that are susceptible to vancomycin include *Clostridia* (including *C. difficile*), *Corynebacterium, Bacillus anthracis, Listeria monocytogenes, Actinomyces* species, and lactobacilli.

Resistance

During the first 30 years of vancomycin use, the development of resistance was not a serious clinical problem. In the last 10 years, however, some resistance has developed. In most cases, resistance to vancomycin is due to the production of a new cell wall component that prevents the drug from binding to the wall. Resistance to vancomycin is reported for *Enterococcus faecalis* due to plasmid-mediated production of a protein that blocks vancomycin from binding to its normal receptor.

Pharmacokinetics

Vancomycin is not absorbed from the GI tract and is irritating if given by IM injection. Therefore, vancomycin is administered by IV, except when it is given orally for the treatment of *Clostridium difficile*, in which case the intent is not to have the drug absorbed. Vancomycin is not metabolized. It is eliminated by glomerular filtration and its dosage is reduced in patients with impaired renal function.

Uses

Vancomycin should be used only in serious gram-positive infections that are not treatable with other antibiotics. It is recommended for serious methicillin-sensitive staphylococcal infections in patients who cannot take a penicillin or cephalosporin (eg, immediate-type hypersensitivity—see Chapter 28) or who have not responded to these drugs.

Vancomycin is the drug of choice for serious infections caused by methicillin-resistant *S. aureus* (MRSA) and coagulase-negative staphylococci, including methicillin-resistant *S. epidermidis* (MRSE). Often, the addition of other drugs (eg, rifampicin, gentamicin) to a vancomycin regimen increases the rate of response.

Vancomycin with gentamicin or streptomycin (for susceptible strains) is used for enterococcal endocarditis in penicillin-allergic patients. IV vancomycin is used for prophylaxis of infective endocarditis in high-risk patients who are allergic to penicillins and are undergoing dental or certain other surgical procedures.

Oral vancomycin is the drug of choice for the treatment of confirmed antibiotic-associated pseudomembranous colitis caused by *Clostridium difficile*.

Adverse Effects

Vancomycin's most common adverse effect is called "red neck" or the "red-man" syndrome. This is a nonimmunologic, dose-dependent, glycopeptide-induced anaphylactoid reaction, characterized by one or more of the following:

- Erythematous macular rash involving the face, neck, upper torso, back, and arms
- Flushing
- Pruritus; pain and muscle spasm in the chest
- Tachycardia
- Hypotension

The exact mechanism of this reaction is unknown. It occurs coincident with an increase in plasma histamine. Pretreatment with antihistamines is effective in preventing this reaction.

NITROFURANTOIN

Actions

Nitrofurantoin's mechanism of action is unclear. The drug inhibits a variety of enzyme systems in bacteria and is active against common urinary pathogens.

Antibacterial Spectrum

Most strains of *Escherichia coli* are susceptible. About two-thirds of other coliform strains are susceptible. *Staphylococcus aureus, Staphylococcus saprophyticus*, and enterococci (*Enterococcus faecalis*) are also susceptible.

Resistance

Susceptible bacteria do not readily develop resistance to nitrofurantoin during therapy.

Pharmacokinetics

Nitrofurantoin is well absorbed from the upper small intestine and is concentrated in the urine. Because nitrofurantoin is associated with a high incidence of GI irritation when it is absorbed quickly (see Adverse Effects below), it is now formulated in large crystals that dissolve slowly and produce less GI intolerance.

Uses

Nitrofurantoin is used to treat urinary tract infections (eg, pyelonephritis, pyelitis, cystitis) that are due to susceptible strains of *E. coli,* enterococci, *S. aureus,* and certain susceptible strains of *Klebsiella, Enterobacter*, and *Proteus* species.

Adverse Effects

GI irritation is the most common adverse effect of nitrofurantoin. Symptoms include anorexia, nausea, and vomiting; diarrhea and abdominal pain occur less frequently. These effects have been partially overcome by increasing the crystal size of the drug and delaying the rate at which nitrofurantoin is absorbed.

Nitrofurantoin can cause allergic reactions including rashes, urticaria, angioneurotic edema, eosinophilia, and fever. Nitrofurantoin can also cause an acute pulmonary reaction, characterized by fever, myalgia, dyspnea, pulmonary infiltration, and pleural effusion.

Nitrofurantoin can also produce a second type of pulmonary reaction involving pneumonic complications and characterized by shortness of breath on exertion and cough.

A sensorimotor peripheral neuropathy has been associated with nitrofurantoin, and is seen most often in patients with impaired renal function.

Nitrofurantoin has also been reported to produce megaloblastic anemia and cholestasis. In patients deficient in glucose-6-phosphate dehydrogenase, the drug can produce hemolysis.

IMIPENEM PLUS CILASTATIN

Actions

Imipenem is a beta-lactam bactericidal antibiotic that inhibits cell wall synthesis in aerobic and anaerobic gram-positive and gram-negative bacteria. It is metabolized to inactive potentially nephrotoxic derivatives by a dihydropeptidase enzyme located in the brush border of the proximal renal tubules. Because of this, only very low concentrations of imipenem can be found in the urine.

Cilastatin blocks the metabolism and inactivation of imipenem in the kidney. By combining cilastatin with imipenem, it is possible to attain antibacterial concentrations of imipenem in the urine.

Antibacterial Spectrum

Imipenem has a wide spectrum of activity. Most aerobic and anaerobic gram-positive and gram-negative species are susceptible. Imipenem owes its activity to 3 major factors:

1. It readily penetrates the cell wall of gram-positive and gram-negative bacteria.
2. It is highly resistant to the activity of most beta-lactamases, whether they are of plasmid or chromosomal origin.
3. It preferentially binds to a critical penicillin-binding protein, PBP-2.

Uses

Neither imipenem nor cilastatin is appreciably absorbed from the GI tract; therefore, they must be injected. The combination of imipenem and cilastatin is used to treat serious infections caused by sensitive bacteria.

Lower respiratory tract infections, urinary tract infections, intra-abdominal and gynecologic infections, and septicemia caused by susceptible bacteria may be treated with imipenem plus cilastatin.

Endocarditis caused by *Staphylococcus aureus* may also be treated with the combination, as can bone, joint, and skin-structure infections produced by susceptible bacteria.

Adverse Effects

The combination of imipenem and cilastatin is generally well tolerated. The most common adverse effects include nausea, diarrhea, and vomiting. However, imipenem plus cilastatin can produce severe allergic reactions. Therefore, this combination should be administered with caution to any patient who has demonstrated some form of allergy, particularly to structurally related drugs (eg, penicillins, cephalosporins). If an allergic reaction occurs to imipenem plus cilastatin, stop the drug. Serious hypersensitivity reactions may require epinephrine and other emergency measures.

Drugs for Systemic Fungal Infections

33

Pharmacotherapy Of Systemic Fungal Infections

Systemic fungal infections constitute a major therapeutic problem and can have a significant fatality rate. Systemic opportunistic infections occur commonly in debilitated and immunosuppressed patients. The more common infections include candidiasis, aspergillosis, cryptococcosis, and phycomycosis.

The treatment of systemic fungal infections is unsatisfactory. Only a limited number of drugs are presently available, and their use is often associated with severe adverse effects. Their use is further complicated by the fact that patients with systemic mycotic infections may be seriously ill with other diseases. Although antibiotics or antibacterials are sometimes used to treat systemic mycotic infections (eg, penicillin G; erythromycin; a cephalosporin, tetracycline, or clindamycin for actinomycosis; a sulfonamide, erythromycin, or tetracycline for nocardiosis), the number of fungal infections that respond to antibiotic/antibacterial therapy is limited. Most systemic mycotic infections require treatment with drugs that were specifically designed to interfere with various aspects of fungal metabolism. These drugs are presented below.

AMPHOTERICIN B

Actions

Amphotericin B owes its fungistatic activity to its ability to interact with fungal membrane sterol ergosterol and increase membrane permeability. Small molecules leak from sensitive fungal cells and amino acid uptake is impaired. Amphotericin B does not affect bacteria, with the exception of *Mycoplasma*, because bacterial cell membranes do not contain sterols. Mammalian cells do contain sterols, and this partly explains amphotericin B's human toxicity.

Antifungal Spectrum

Amphotericin B has a broad spectrum of activity. It is effective against *Cryptococcus neoformans*, *Histoplasma capsulatum*, *Coccidioides immitis*, *Blastomyces dermatitidis*, and *Sporothrix schenckii*.

Pharmacokinetics

Because amphotericin B is poorly absorbed from the GI tract, it must be administered by IV. Amphotericin B has an initial half-life of 24 hours. However, because it is extensively stored in body tissues, the drug has a second half-life of 15 days. Although amphotericin B crosses the blood-brain barrier, its concentration in the CSF is lower than its level in blood. Its major route of excretion is extrarenal.

Uses

Amphotericin B is used to treat patients with progressive, potentially fatal disseminated mycotic infections. It can be used to treat opportunistic infections in immunosuppressed patients caused by *Candida*, *Cryptococcus*, and *Torulopsis*. Because amphotericin B does not diffuse well into the CSF, intrathecal administration may be required for CNS infections.

Adverse Effects

Amphotericin B must be used with care. The most common early effect is an acute febrile reaction beginning about 2 hours after starting the infusion and peaking approximately 1 hour later.

Amphotericin B can produce a dose-dependent azotemia. Reversible normocytic, normochromic anemia is common with prolonged therapy.

Hypersensitivity reactions are not usual. However, amphotericin B can produce generalized pain, seizures, and anaphylactic shock. It can also cause headache, fever, chills, anorexia, and vomiting.

FLUCYTOSINE

Actions

Flucytosine is a fungistatic structural analogue of cytosine, an essential component in body functions. Once taken up into fungal cells via cytosine permease, flucytosine is deaminated by fungal cytosine deaminase to form fluorouracil (5-FU) and fluorodeoxyuridine monophosphate. Fluorouracil is incorporated into fungal RNA and inhibits protein synthesis.

Antifungal Spectrum

Flucytosine inhibits the growth of *Cryptococcus neoformas, Candida albicans, Torulopsis glabrata, Sporothrix schenckii, Cladosporium* species, and *Phialophora* species, the fungi responsible for chromomycosis. Resistance has been reported to flucytosine. This may reflect a deficiency in the enzymes involved in the transport of the drug into the cytoplasm, or it may be due to a compensatory ability of the organism to increase its rate of pyrimidine synthesis.

Pharmacokinetics

Flucytosine is well absorbed and can be found in the serum 30 minutes after oral administration. It is widely distributed in body fluids and readily crosses the blood-brain barrier to enter the CSF. Because flucytosine is excreted primarily by the kidneys, its dosage schedule must be modified in patients with impaired renal function. Flucytosine has a half-life of 3 to 5 hours.

Uses

Flucytosine is used to treat serious infections caused by susceptible strains of *Candida* or *Cryptococcus*, or both. Flucytosine passes easily into the CSF and enters the aqueous humor and bronchial secretions in concentrations adequate to inhibit sensitive fungi. It has effectively treated septicemia, endocarditis, and urinary tract infections caused by *Candida*, as well as meningitis and pulmonary infections caused by *Cryptococcus*. Other uses for flucytosine include the treatment of chromomycosis caused by *Fonsecaea pedrosoi, Cladosporium carrioni,* and *Phialophora verrucosa*. Because resistance may develop during therapy, flucytosine is usually combined with amphotericin B.

Adverse Effects

Flucytosine's principal adverse effects are reversible neutropenia, together with occasional thrombocytopenia. Flucytosine can also cause nausea, eosinophilia, and skin rashes. It is also capable of producing reversible hepatic dysfunction. Patients sometimes experience confusion, hallucinations, headache, and vertigo. A few cases of irreversible bone marrow failure have been reported. Flucytosine's metabolite, fluorodeoxyuridine monophosphate, (see Actions above) inhibits DNA synthesis and is probably responsible for bone marrow depression. Patients with a limited bone marrow reserve, such as individuals receiving cytotoxic drug treatment, may be prone to develop hematologic adverse effects when treated with flucytosine.

3. AZOLE ANTIFUNGAL DRUGS

Fluconazole, Itraconazole, Ketoconazole

Actions

Fluconazole and itraconazole are called **triazoles** because they contain three nitrogens in an azole ring.

Ketoconazole is classified as an **imidazole** because it contains two nitrogens in an azole ring.

All azole antifungal drugs bind to the heme iron of cytochrome P-450 and inhibit the demethylation of 14-alpha-methyl-sterols to ergosterol. Ergosterol is the main sterol in the fungal cell membrane. Inhibiting its formation alters the permeability of the fungal cell membrane. Both fluconazole and itraconazole have greater specificity for fungal cytochrome P-450 than for the mammalian cytochrome. This may account for the relatively low toxicity of the triazoles compared with the imidazoles.

Antifungal Spectra

Fluconazole has broad-spectrum activity and is effective in the treatment of aspergillosis, blastomycosis, candidiasis, cryptococcosis, and histoplasmosis.

Itraconazole has an antifungal spectrum similar to that of ketoconazole (see below), except that it is also active against *Aspergillus* species and *Sporothrix schenckii*.

Ketoconazole is effective against a variety of fungi and yeasts, including *Blastomyces dermatitidis*, *Candida*, *Coccidioides immitis*, *Histoplasma capsulatum*, and dermatophytes.

Pharmacokinetics

Fluconazole, with an oral bioavailability of over 90%, can be given orally or by IV. Fluconazole penetrates all body tissues and fluids, and its apparent volume of distribution approximates that of the total body water. Its terminal half-life is approximately 30 hours, allowing for once-daily dosing. Because fluconazole's rate of elimination decreases as kidney function falls, its dosage should be reduced in patients with renal impairment.

Itraconazole's oral absorption is variable and requires a low gastric pH. Food enhances itraconazole absorption. The drug is concentrated in lipophilic tissues. Itraconazole is metabolized by the liver and excreted in the bile and has a plasma half-life of 30 to 35 hours after multiple doses.

Ketoconazole is well absorbed from the GI tract, but it is best absorbed at low pH values. Drugs that increase gastric pH reduce ketoconazole absorption. Ketoconazole is distributed widely throughout the tissues and tissue fluids but does not reach therapeutic concentrations in the CNS unless high doses are given. The drug is inactivated in the liver and excreted in the bile and urine. Its plasma half-life is 8 hours.

Uses

Fluconazole is used to treat oropharyngeal and esophageal candidiasis. It is also effective for the treatment of serious systemic candidal infections, including urinary tract infections, peritonitis, and pneumonitis. Fluconazole is also indicated for the treatment of cryptococcal meningitis. It is also used to prevent cryptococcal meningitis recurrence in patients with AIDS. Oral fluconazole has also been approved for the treatment of vaginal candidiasis.

Itraconazole is indicated for the treatment of the following infections in normal, predisposed, or immunocompromised patients: invasive and noninvasive pulmonary aspergillosis, oral/esophageal candidiasis, chronic pulmonary histoplasmosis, cutaneous and lymphatic sporotrichosis, paracoccidioidomycosis, chromomycosis, and blastomycosis.

Ketoconazole is used to treat serious life-threatening systemic fungal infections in normal, predisposed, or immunocompromised patients for whom alternative therapy is considered inappropriate or has been unsuccessful. This includes systemic candidiasis, chronic mucocutaneous candidiasis, coccidioidomycosis and paracoccidioidomycosis, histoplasmosis, and chromomycosis. Ketoconazole is not indicated in the treatment of CNS fungal infections because it poorly penetrates the CNS.

Adverse Effects

Fluconazole's most serious adverse effects appear to be exfoliative skin disorders and hepatic necrosis. Immunocompromised patients (especially those with AIDS) who develop rashes during treatment with fluconazole should be monitored carefully. If lesions progress, fluconazole should be stopped. Patients with baseline abnormal liver function tests, and those who develop abnormal liver function tests during fluconazole therapy, should be monitored for the development of more severe hepatic injury. Other adverse effects of fluconazole include nausea, headache, skin rash, vomiting, abdominal pain, and diarrhea.

Itraconazole's most common adverse effects involve the GI tract, including nausea. These are followed by dermatologic reactions (rash and pruritus), headache, and effects involving the respiratory system. For therapy longer than 30 days, liver function should be monitored.

Ketoconazole's most common adverse effects are nausea and pruritus. Patients may also experience headache, dizziness, abdominal pain, constipation, diarrhea, somnolence, and nervousness. Concern is greatest for possible hepatotoxic effects. Cases of fatal massive hepatic necrosis have been reported and liver function should be monitored periodically. Ketoconazole can block adrenal steroid synthesis. Approximately 10% of men experience gynecomastia.

34

Drugs for the Treatment of Viral Infections

Characteristics of Viruses and Difficulties in Developing Selective Antiviral Drugs

Viruses are among the simplest living organisms. Composed of a protein coat and one or more strands of a linear or helical nucleic acid core, (either DNA or RNA), a mature virus can exist outside a host cell and still retain its infective properties. However, to reproduce, the virus must enter the host cell, take over the cell's mechanism for nucleic acid and protein synthesis, and direct the host cell to make new viral particles. Viruses are essentially intracellular parasites that utilize many of the biochemical mechanisms and products of the host cell to sustain their viability. This makes it difficult to find a drug that is selective for the virus that does not interfere with host cell function.

This chapter will be divided into two parts:

- Drugs for the treatment of AIDS
- Drugs for the treatment of some other common viral infections

B. DRUGS FOR THE TREATMENT OF AIDS

Acquired immunodeficiency syndrome (AIDS) is caused by a retrovirus called the human immunodeficiency virus (HIV). Retroviruses are a subgroup of RNA viruses which, in order to replicate, must first *"reverse transcribe"* their RNA genome into DNA. Once in the form of DNA, the viral genome is incorporated into the host cell genome, allowing it to take full advantage of the host cell's transcription/translation machinery for the purpose of replication. Anti-AIDS drugs are used to:

1. attack the virus (anti-HIV drugs), or
2. to treat infections that have arisen as a result of the host's reduced immune response (supportive therapy).

1. Anti-HIV Drugs

Multiplication of HIV

HIV possesses an envelope glycoprotein (gp120) with a high affinity for the CD4 receptor on host T-helper cells. As a result, the HIV binds to the T cell and fuses with the lymphocyte surface membrane. Thereafter, the virus loses its coat and releases its RNA core and reverse transcriptase enzyme into the host cell cytoplasm (Figures 34–1 and 34–2). The HIV reverse transcriptase copies the RNA message, producing a double-stranded proviral DNA, which enters the host cell nucleus and becomes incorporated into the host chromosomal DNA. The incorporated viral DNA may remain dormant or, on activation, produce viral messenger RNA (mRNA). The viral mRNA codes for proteins that are important in viral replication. Glycoproteins will then envelop the RNA genome, resulting in the production of infectious viral particles. The completed viral particles are then released to infect other host cells.

Actions of Anti-HIV Drugs

Three classes of antiviral drugs are currently used to treat HIV infections:

- Nucleoside and Nucleoside Analogue Reverse Transcriptase Inhibitors (**NRTIs**)
- Non-nucleoside Analogue Reverse Transcriptase Inhibitors (**NNRTIs**)
- Protease Inhibitors (**PIs**)

Table 34–1 lists some currently available NRTIs, NNRTIs, and PIs.

Table 34–1
Currently Available Anti-HIV Drugs

NRTI	NNRTI	PI
Abacavir	Delaviridine	Indinavir
Didanosine	Efavirenz	Nelfinavir
Lamivudine	Nevirapine	Ritonavir
Stavudine		Saquinavir
Zalcitabine		
Zidovudine		

NRTI = nucleoside reverse transcriptase inhibitor; NNRTI = non-nucleoside reverse transcriptase inhibitor; PI = protease inhibitor.

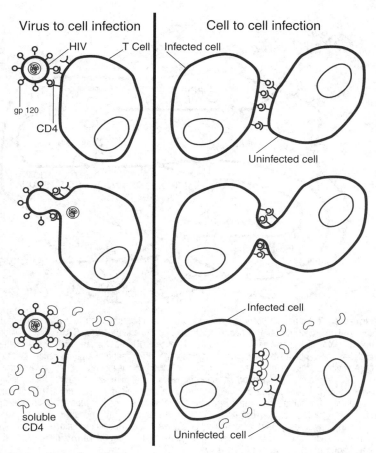

Figure 34–1 HIV infective mechanism. Virus to cell infection (upper left): The gp120 knob-like surface protein contacts the CD4 receptor on T lymphocytes or other cells. The virus fuses with the cell and RNA is uncoated (middle left). If soluble CD4 molecules are present, they can bind to the gp120 projections on the HIV and prevent infection of the host cell (lower left). Cell to cell infection: Once a cell is infected, it can infect noninfected cells by fusion of processed surface gp120 with CD4 receptors of the uninfected cells (upper right). By fusion of infected and multiple noninfected cells, a multinucleated giant cell can be produced (middle right). If soluble CD4 proteins exist, cell-to-cell fusion could be prevented (lower right). HIV = human immunodeficiency virus; gp = glycoprotein; RNA = ribonucleic acid. (After Van Dyke K. Drugs used in acquired immunodeficiency syndrome. In: Craig CR, Stitzel RE, editors. Modern pharmacology. 4th ed. New York: Little Brown; 1994.)

These drugs target two events in the HIV replication cycle:

1. Reverse transcription of the viral RNA into double-stranded proviral DNA by the viral reverse transcriptase (**NRTIs and NNRTIs**)
2. Processing of the viral precursor protein by viral protease (ie, assembly of the viral particles) (**PIs**)

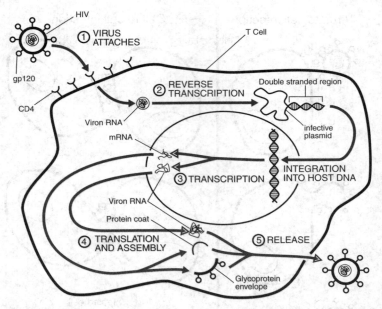

Figure 34–2 Steps that occur in viral infection and replication. Step 1: HIV infection of a T cell. The gp120 viral knob attaches to a CD4 lymphocyte receptor. Step 2: HIV viral RNA produces a DNA copy using reverse transcriptase. The linear DNA has long terminal repeats at each end that are complementary, and can participate in the formation of a partly double-stranded DNA plasmid. This infective plasmid migrates into the nucleus of the host cell and integrates into its DNA. Step 3: Transcription. At some point, host DNA, RNA, and protein synthesis is shut off and viral RNA and protein synthesis is turned on, resulting in transcription of RNA. Step 4: Translation. Translation into protein and assembly of viral particles surrounded by an envelope glycoprotein now occur. Step 5: Release of the completed virus. HIV = human immunodeficiency virus; gp = glycoprotein; RNA = ribonucleic acid; DNA = deoxyribonucleic acid. (After Van Dyke K. Drugs used in acquired immunodeficiency syndrome. In: Craig CR, Stitzel RE, editors. Modern Pharmacology. 4th ed. New York: Little Brown; 1994.)

Uses

Anti-HIV drugs are used in combination in order to delay the development of drug resistance.

- **Initial therapy for patients with a high viral load usually involves two NRTIs plus a PI.**
  - ◆ In patients who can comply with these regimens, dramatic reductions in viral load are seen.
  - ◆ The disadvantage of starting with a regimen that uses agents from more than one class is that when drug failure eventually occurs, resistance to several classes of drugs can exist, thereby limiting the choices available for rescue therapy.
- **The alternative approach for initial therapy is using only NRTI drugs.**

- ◆ This approach has the advantage of reserving the potent PI class or the NNRTI class as key components for future therapy.
- ◆ However, combinations containing three NRTI drugs have not been as potent as regimens containing two NRTIs and one PI. As a result, triple NRTI combinations have only been used as initial therapy in patients who present with a low to moderate viral load.
- ◆ Published data appear to demonstrate that replacing a PI with abacavir in combination with two other NRTIs (lamivudine and zidovudine) does not result in a loss of clinical efficacy. This protocol could save a PI for the day when resistance to NRTI therapy develops.

- **For patients with previous exposure to antiretroviral therapy, treatment should include:**
  - ◆ the addition of at least two new agents, or
  - ◆ a switch to a completely new triple therapy that should ideally have no overlapping resistance or toxicity with previously available therapy.

Adverse Effects

All anti-HIV drugs have the potential to produce severe adverse effects.

NRTIs frequently produce nausea, abdominal pain, diarrhea, headache, insomnia, myalgia, and peripheral neuropathy. Hypersensitivity reactions are a potential problem with some NRTIs.

NNRTIs can produce rash, nausea, fatigue, somnolence, headache, and hepatotoxicity. Nevirapine has also been reported to produce Stevens-Johnson syndrome.

PIs can also produce diarrhea, abdominal discomfort, and nausea. It is their ability to increase triglycerides, produce diabetes, and induce lipodystrophies that frequently causes the greatest concern because they can alert others to the HIV status of the patient. Some PIs have also been reported to produce allergic reactions, including urticaria, mild skin eruptions, bronchospasm, and angioedema. Hepatic transaminase elevations, clinical hepatitis, and jaundice have also been reported with PIs. Nephrolithiasis is an adverse effect of indinavir.

2. Supportive Therapy

People with AIDS are susceptible to *opportunistic infections* (ie, infections that would not normally be found in patients with normal defence mechanisms). The appropriate use of antibiotics, antifungals, and antivirals can significantly prolong life in HIV-infected individuals. Table 34–2 summarizes the management of selected HIV-associated infections.

Many of the drugs used as supportive therapy in AIDS patients are described elsewhere. Three drugs not otherwise presented are summarized here.

Foscarnet Sodium

Actions

Foscarnet inhibits the DNA polymerase of human herpes viruses and the reverse transcriptase of HIV at a different site from nucleoside analogues, such as ganciclovir, acyclovir, or zidovudine. In vitro, foscarnet inhibits replication of cytomegalovirus (CMV), herpes simplex (HSV) 1 and 2, varicella zoster (VZV), and HIV at concentrations easily achieved with parenteral therapy.

Uses

Foscarnet is administered by IV to treat CMV retinitis in patients with AIDS. It can also be used to treat ganciclovir-resistant CMV infections. Fos-

Table 34–2
Management of Selected HIV-Associated Infections

Infection	Treatment
Candida species • Mucosal candidal infections • Esophageal candidiasis • Severe discomfort or esophageal disease requires systemic therapy	Thrush topical treatment • Nystatin suspension swished and swallowed, or vaginal tablet, sucked • Clotrimazole vaginal tablet sucked or clotrimazole troche Vaginal infection • Miconazole or clotrimazole vaginal cream or suppository Systemic oral therapy • Fluconazole is first choice • Ketoconazole or itraconazole are alternatives Esophageal disease • Fluconazole or amphotericin B
Cryptococcus neoformans • Major cause of meningitis in later stages of HIV infection (in 10% of AIDS patients) • Ongoing prophylactic therapy required after treatment of acute infection	Induction therapy • Amphotericin B ± flucytosine for 2 weeks, then completion of 12-week course with fluconazole Maintenance therapy • Fluconazole or amphotericin B weekly

Continued

Table 34–2
Management of Selected HIV-Associated Infections—Continued

Infection	Treatment
Cytomegalovirus (CMV) • Retinitis with visual disturbances is most common manifestation • Enteritis, colitis, pneumonitis, encephalitis, myelitis, and neuritis can also occur • Prognosis is poor without therapy • Life-long maintenance therapy required after initial therapy for CMV retinitis	Induction therapy • Ganciclovir or foscarnet Maintenance therapy • Ganciclovir or foscarnet
Mycobacterium avium complex (MAC) • Symptoms: fever, weight loss, fatigue, and night sweats either alone or with diarrhea, anemia, lymphadenopathy, hepatitis	Multidrug regimens • Usually include clarithromycin or azithromycin + ethambutol ± 1–3 additional drugs (such as rifampin or rifabutin, ciprofloxacin, clofazimine, and amikacin)
Pneumocystis carinii • Primary cause of pneumonia in HIV-positive patients with CD4 < 200 cells/mm^2 • All patients at risk should receive prophylaxis • Commonly presents as persistent fever with progressive shortness of breath and cough, often with normal chest radiograph	Standard therapy • Cotrimoxazole, or pentamidine, or dapsone + trimethoprim Other therapies • Atovaquone, clindamycin + primaquine, trimetrexate + folinic acid Prednisone • Addition of prednisone in severe PCP decreases morbidity and side effects of cotrimoxazole
Toxoplasma gondii • Up to 50% of HIV-positive patients with antibodies to this parasite will develop toxoplasma encephalitis as CD4 fall below 200 cells/mm^3 • Most commonly presents as fever with focal neurologic signs	Standard Therapy • Pyrimethamine + folinic acid + sulfadiazine Alternatives • Pyrimethamine + folinic acid + (clindamycin or azithromycin), or (clarithromycin, dapsone, or atovaquone) Maintenance therapy • Pyrimethamine + sulfadiazine + folinic acid, or pyrimethamine + clindamycin + folinic acid

HIV = human immunodeficiency virus; PCP = *Pneumocystis carinii* pneumonia. After Gregson DB. Opportunistic infections in HIV-positive patients. In: Therapeutic Choices, Canadian Pharmacists Association. 3rd ed., 2000. p. 798–809.

carnet appears to be the drug of choice for the treatment of acyclovir-resistant HSV and VZV infections.

Adverse Effects

Nephrotoxicity is the most common dose-limiting adverse effect of foscarnet. Foscarnet binds divalent metal ions, such as calcium. Metabolic abnormalities (eg, hypocalcemia, hypomagnesemia, hypophosphatemia), which are all apparently related to this effect, occur commonly. Foscarnet can also produce hypokalemia. High maintenance doses of foscarnet cause a decrease in ionized calcium (with normal total serum calcium concentrations) that may cause neurologic and cardiac toxicity. Other adverse effects include nausea, seizures, neutropenia, neuropathy, arrhythmia, nephrogenic diabetes insipidus, and penile ulcers.

Ganciclovir

Actions, Uses, and Adverse Effects

Ganciclovir is a synthetic nucleoside analogue that inhibits the replication of herpes viruses. Ganciclovir is used to treat CMV retinitis in immuno-compromised individuals, such as patients with AIDS, those with iatrogenic immunosuppression secondary to organ transplantation, or those undergoing chemotherapy for neoplasia. Ganciclovir's most frequent adverse effects involve the hematopoietic system (eg, neutropenia and thrombocytopenia).

Pentamidine

Actions, Uses, and Adverse Effects

Pneumocystis carinii pneumonia (PCP) occurs in approximately 80% of AIDS patients and is a significant cause of death. Current therapies for PCP are cotrimoxazole (Chapter 32) and parenteral pentamidine. Either therapy is effective but adverse effects limit their potential. Pentamidine should be given parenterally only in a hospital with facilities to monitor blood glucose, blood counts, and renal and hepatic function. Fatalities due to severe hypotension, hypoglycemia, and cardiac arrhythmias have been reported in patients treated with parenteral pentamidine. Profound severe hypotension may result after a single dose.

Aerosolized pentamidine isethionate once a month is effective in preventing recurrence of PCP in AIDS patients.

DRUGS FOR THE TREATMENT OF SOME OTHER COMMON VIRAL INFECTIONS

Acyclovir

Actions

Acyclovir is metabolized to acyclovir triphosphate, which inhibits DNA polymerase and viral multiplication in herpes simplex types 1 and 2, varicella zoster, herpes simiae (B virus), and Epstein-Barr virus.

Uses

When injected, acyclovir is used to treat initial and recurrent mucosal and cutaneous herpes simplex infections in immunocompromised adults and children. Injectable acyclovir is also used for severe initial episodes of herpes simplex infections in patients who may not be immunocompromised.

Oral acyclovir may be used in the treatment of an initial episode of herpes genitalis and the suppression of unusually frequent recurrences of herpes genitalis.

Acyclovir is applied topically for management of initial episodes of genital herpes simplex infections. The topical preparation is also used for the management of non-life-threatening cutaneous herpes simplex viral infections in immunocompromised patients.

Adverse Effects

Acyclovir appears to be a relatively safe drug, but a few patients have experienced delirium. A causal relationship to acyclovir has not been established. Other reported adverse effects include inflammation and/or phlebitis at the injection site, and diaphoresis, hematuria, hypotension, headache, and nausea. Hives have been reported in some patients after acyclovir injection.

Oral acyclovir may produce nausea and vomiting, headache, diarrhea, skin rash, vertigo, and arthralgia.

Topical acyclovir may produce discomfort.

Amantadine

Actions and Uses

Amantadine may inhibit penetration of influenza A viruses into the host cell or reduce the uncoating of those viruses that do penetrate the cell.

Amantadine is used in the prevention and treatment of respiratory infections caused by influenza A virus strains. It may have its greatest value in patients at high risk of developing influenza because of underlying disease, such as the elderly in hospitals or nursing homes. Amantadine does not interfere with immunization, and patients may receive amantadine while waiting for the effects of immunization to develop. If used to treat an influenza A virus infection, amantadine must be started within 48 hours of the onset of symptoms.

Adverse Effects

Amantadine is generally well tolerated. The more important adverse effects are orthostatic hypotensive episodes, congestive heart failure, depression, psychosis, and urinary retention.

Idoxuridine

Actions and Uses

Idoxuridine is incorporated into viral DNA, destabilizing the nucleic acid and altering viral protein synthesis. Ophthalmic idoxuridine is used topically to treat herpes simplex keratitis. Epithelial infections, especially initial attacks, characterized by the presence of a dendritic figure, are highly responsive to idoxuridine. Infections located in the stroma have shown a less favorable response. In recurrent cases, idoxuridine will often control the current episode of the viral infection, but scarring from previous infections will not be corrected.

Adverse Effects

Idoxuridine can cause clouding of the cornea and small defects in the corneal epithelium. It may also cause local irritation, itching, mild edema, and photophobia.

Ribavirin

Actions and Uses

Ribavirin is active against the respiratory syncytial (RS) virus. Its mechanism of action is not known. Ribavirin is approved only for lower respiratory tract infections due to the RS virus. Ribavirin aerosol treatment must be accompanied by (and does not replace) standard supportive respiratory and fluid management for infants and children with severe respiratory tract infections.

Adverse Effects

Serious adverse effects that have occurred during ribavirin therapy have included worsening of respiratory status, bacterial pneumonia, and pneumothorax. It is not clear whether these effects are related to the use of ribavirin.

Trifluridine

Actions and Uses

Trifluridine is phosphorylated by a cellular thymidine kinase to its nucleotide monophosphate. Trifluridine monophosphate and its metabolites inhibit the following DNA viruses: herpes simplex types 1 and 2, varicella zoster, adenovirus, and vaccinia virus. Trifluridine is approved for the treatment of primary keratoconjunctivitis and recurrent epithelial keratitis due to herpes simplex viruses types 1 and 2.

Adverse Effects

The most common adverse effects are burning on instillation and superficial punctate keratitis.

Inhibitors of Influenza Virus Neuraminidase (Oseltamivir and Zanamivir)

Actions and Uses

Oseltamivir and zanamivir are potent selective inhibitors of neuraminidase, the influenza virus surface enzyme that aids the release of newly formed virus particles from infected cells. Neuraminidase may also facilitate access of the influenza virus through mucus to epithelial cell surfaces, enabling the virus to infect other cells. By inhibiting the action of neuraminidase, oseltamivir and zanamivir reduce the spread of influenza A and B viruses by suppressing the release of infectious virions from the epithelial cells of the respiratory tract.

Oseltamivir is converted to its active metabolite oseltamivir carboxylate following oral administration. Oseltamivir is approved for the treatment of uncomplicated illness due to influenza infection in adults who have been symptomatic for no more than 2 days.

Zanamivir is administered as a dry powder by oral inhalation, allowing high concentrations of the drug to act extracellularly to inhibit viral neuraminidase. Zanamivir is approved for the treatment of uncomplicated acute illness due to influenza virus in patients 12 years and older, who have been symptomatic for no more than 2 days.

Adverse Effects

Oseltamivir's most frequent adverse effects in clinical trials were nausea and vomiting. Events were transient and generally occurred with first dosing.

Zanamivir is well tolerated when inhaled by young adults. In clinical studies in young adults, the incidence of adverse effects reported was similar in the zanamivir and placebo groups.

35

Anticancer Drugs (Antineoplastic Drugs)

GENERAL COMMENTS

Goal of Cancer Chemotherapy

The goal of cancer chemotherapy is to kill malignant tumor cells and spare host cells. This is called **selective toxicity**. Selective toxicity forms the basis of all antibiotic, antifungal, and antiviral therapy previously presented. However, selective toxicity is relatively easy to achieve in anti-infective therapy because mammalian cells and bacterial cells, for example, differ markedly in their structure and metabolic processes. Selective chemotherapy is not, however, easy to achieve in cancer treatment because normal and malignant cells often do not differ markedly. Therefore, it is virtually impossible to kill large numbers of cancer cells without destroying at least some normal cells.

Cells Killed by Anticancer Drugs

Anticancer drugs suppress all proliferating cells, both normal and neoplastic. This effect accounts for their major toxicities on such rapidly dividing cells as bone marrow, GI and germinal epithelia, hair follicles, and lymphoid organs. Thus, successful anticancer therapy is defined differently than successful anti-infective treatment. Successful antineoplastic treatment depends on killing malignant tumor cells with doses of anticancer drugs that allow recovery of normal proliferating cells. To understand how this can be achieved, it is important to review the relationship of cellular growth fraction to cancer chemotherapy.

289

RELATIONSHIP OF GROWTH FRACTION TO SUCCESS OF CHEMOTHERAPY

The Cell Cycle

Figure 35–1 presents the cell cycle. Every cell that divides passes through specific phases before undergoing mitosis.

- During the synthesis (S) phase, lasting from 6 to 50 hours, DNA synthesis increases and chromosomal material doubles.
- Thereafter, the cell proceeds through the G_2 phase, lasting about 6 hours, during which time a series of biochemical events occur that prepare the cell for mitosis.
- After mitosis (the M phase), new cells enter the G_1 phase. Depending on the cells involved, G_1 may last minutes or years.
- Cell progressing through G_1, S, G_2. and mitosis are said to be **"in cycle."** Cells not actively dividing are said to be in the G_0 phase.

Growth Fraction

Every tissue, whether normal or neoplastic, has a portion of its cells that are not actively dividing. They can be found side by side with dividing cells. The number of cells in cycle divided by the total number of cells in the tissue is the **growth fraction**. The growth fraction does not remain constant. Larger tumors have smaller growth fractions. If the size of the tumor is reduced,

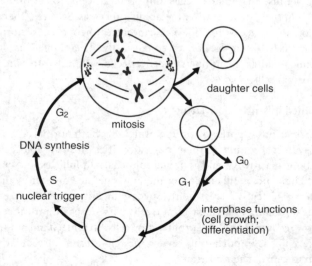

Figure 35–1 The cell cycle.

either by surgery, radiation, or antineoplastic drugs, more resting cells begin to cycle.

Cells in cycle ⇌ Resting cells

Relative Efficacy of Anticancer Drugs Against Cells in Cycle Versus Resting Cells

Anticancer drugs are more effective against proliferating cells than cells in G_0 because antineoplastic agents usually kill cells by disrupting either DNA synthesis or mitosis, functions that occur only in proliferating cells. Thus, as a general rule, **antineoplastic drugs are much more toxic to tissues that have a high growth fraction than to tissues whose growth fraction is low.**

- Solid tumors (eg, those of the lung, breast, stomach, colon, and rectum) have a low growth fraction and often respond poorly to anticancer drugs.
- Disseminated tumors (eg, leukemias and lymphomas) have a high growth fraction and generally respond well to antineoplastic drugs.

Combination Chemotherapy

Cancer chemotherapy that uses a combination of drugs is considerably more effective than therapy with just one drug. The benefits of combination therapy are:

(a) suppression of drug resistance,
(b) enhancement of therapeutic effects, and
(c) reduced injury to normal cells.

If several drugs are selected with different mechanisms of action, drug resistance occurs less frequently and more malignant cells are killed.

Because *PDQ Pharmacology* is a small book, intended to assist students grasp the concepts that underlie the use of groups of drugs, space does not allow a discussion of the merits of the various combinations of anticancer drugs used to treat each disease. Suffice it to say that most cancers are routinely treated with a combination or "cocktail" of several antineoplastics.

DRUG RESISTANCE

Explanations for Resistance to Anticancer Drugs

Some patients treated with cancer chemotherapy fail to respond from the outset. In such patients, their cancers are resistant to drug therapy. Initial drug resistance can be explained by the fact that cancers are not composed of homogeneous cells. Rather, human tumors contain various subpopulations of cells that differ genetically and structurally from one another—some are sensitive to a particular drug, others are not. Given the large number of cells present within most tumors at the time of diagnosis, it seems likely that at least one resistant subpopulation will be present for each individual anticancer drug. Killing of the sensitive cells leads to the proliferation of the resistant. The use of combination chemotherapy, whereby all cells in a tumor may respond to at least one drug, reduces the chance that this form of drug resistance will develop.

Other patients initially respond, and subsequently relapse. For these individuals, their cancers have developed resistance to chemotherapy. Figure 35–2 presents the major mechanisms of cellular resistance to anticancer drugs.

- Resistance to an anticancer drug can develop at its site of action. Resistance develops to methotrexate, for example, because of an alteration in the structure of the target enzyme, dihydrofolate reductase, which results in reduced drug affinity.
- Tumor cells may become resistant to anticancer drugs because they either fail to take up or retain sufficient drug. This type of resistance is called multidrug resistance. It is the major form of resistance shown to anthracyclines, vinca alkaloids, etoposide, paclitaxel, and dactinomycin.

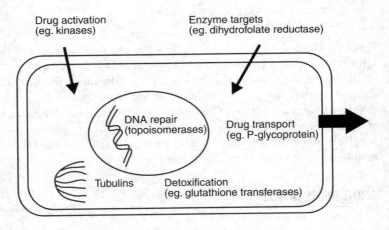

Figure 35–2 Cellular resistance to anticancer drugs. After Sikic BI. The rational basis for cancer chemotherapy. In: Craig CR, Stitzel RE, editors. Modern Pharmacology. 4th ed. Boston: Little Brown; 1994. p. 663–72.

Multidrug resistance results from the production of a high-molecular-weight membrane protein called the P-glycoprotein, which acts to increase the efflux of antineoplastic drugs out of the cells.

- Resistance can develop to alkylating agents because of changes in cell DNA repair capabilities, increases in thiol content (which serves as alternative and benign targets of alklylation), decreases in cell permeability, and increases in glutathione transferase activity. The last phenomenon increases the cellular detoxification of alkylating agents.

- Some drugs must be metabolically activated to function as anticancer agents. These include the antimetabolites 6-fluorouracil and 6-mercaptopurine. These drugs may be ineffective if a tumor is lacking the enzymes required for their activation. The reverse is also true. Some drugs, such as cytarabine and bleomycin, can be metabolically inactivated by resistant tumors.

CLASSIFICATION OF ANTINEOPLASTIC DRUGS

1. Classification Based on Cell Cycle

Cell-Cycle Independent Antineoplastics

Antineoplastics are characterized as cell-cycle independent if they affect cells during any phase of the cycle, including resting or G_0 cells.

Cell-Cycle Dependent Antineoplastics

Anticancer drugs are considered to be cell-cycle dependent if they affect only cells that are actively cycling at the time of exposure to the drug. Antineoplastics may also be phase dependent if one specific phase of the cycle is the principle target of drug action. For example, the vinca alkaloids vinblastine, vincristine, vindesine, and vinorelbine block mitosis and are considered phase-dependent drugs.

2. Classification Based on Mechanism of Action or Source of Drug (Table 35–1)

Alkylating Agents

By definition, alkylating agents introduce alkyl groups into nucleophilic sites on other molecules. Their most important targets are the pyrimidine and purine bases in DNA. These drugs interfere with RNA transcription, thereby inhibiting cell growth and causing death. The degree to which each drug can alkylate DNA correlates well with its cytotoxicity. This interaction

Table 35–1

Classification of Antineoplastic Drugs According to Mechanism of Action or Source of Drug

Classification	Drug
Alkylating agents	Busulphan, Carboplatin, Carmustine (BCNU), Chlorambucil, Cisplatin, Cyclo-phosphamide, Dacarbazine, Ifosfamide, Lomustine (CCNU), Mechlorethamine HCl (Nitrogen Mustard), Melphalan, Streptozocin, Thiotepa
Antimetabolites	Cladribine, Cytarabine (Cytosine Arabinoside), Floxuridine, Fludarabine, Fluorouracil (5-FU), Hydroxyurea, Mercaptopurine (6-MP), Methotrexate (Amethopterin), Thioguanine
Antitumor antibiotics	Bleomycin, Dactinomycin (Actinomycin D), Daunorubicin (Daunomycin), Doxorubicin, Idarubicin, Mitomycin, Pentostatin, Plicamycin (Mithramycin)
Plant-derived products	Docetaxel, Etoposide, Paclitaxel, Teniposide, Vinblastine, Vincristine, Vindesine, Vinorelbine
Hormones and drugs that affect hormone secretion or action	Aminoglutethimide, Buserelin, Flutamide, Goserelin, Leuprolide, Megestrol, Mitotane, Tamoxifen, Testolactone
Miscellaneous antineoplastics	Asparaginase, Procarbazine

also accounts for the mutagenic and carcinogenic properties of the alkylating agents. By attaching to components of DNA molecules, alkylating agents inhibit DNA replication and transcription, leading to cell death.

Antimetabolites

The antimetabolites listed in Table 35–1 are structurally similar to important chemicals in the body. These structural similarities allow antimetabolites to compete with normal body metabolites for vital enzymes. If an antimetabolite replaces a normal metabolite on a vital enzyme, it blocks reactions that are essential to cell function and life.

• Methotrexate is similar in structure to dihydrofolate, a metabolite of folic acid, and it competes with dihydrofolate for binding to the enzyme dihydrofolate reductase. The reduction of dihydrofolate by dihydrofolate reductase is essential in the transfer of single carbon units that are necessary in DNA and purine synthesis. When methotrexate competes successfully with dihydrofolate for binding sites on dihydrofolate reductase, it inhibits DNA and purine synthesis.

- Cytosine, thymine, and uracil are pyrimidines. They are employed in the biosynthesis of DNA and RNA. Cytarabine and 5-FU are two antimetabolites of pyrimidines. Like all pyrimidine antimetabolites, these drugs are metabolized into compounds that are structurally very similar to pyrimidines. Because of this structural similarity, the drugs can replace pyrimidines in key metabolic reactions and cause cell death.

- Adenine, guanine, and hypoxanthine are purines. Purines, like pyrimidines, are used in the synthesis of DNA and RNA. Administering a purine analogue, such as thioguanine, 6-MP, or fludarabine, blocks vital metabolic functions and kills cells.

Antitumor Antibiotics

Bleomycin, dactinomycin, daunorubicin, doxorubicin, idarubicin, mitomycin, and plicamycin are cytotoxic compounds produced by microorganisms. These drugs produce their cytotoxic effects through direct interaction with DNA. Bleomycin, for example, binds to DNA and produces both single- and double-strand breaks and fragmentation of DNA.

Plant-Derived Products

Several important antineoplastics are derived from plants.

- The vinca alkaloids vinblastine, vincristine, vindesine, and vinorelbine are either naturally occurring or semisynthetic products derived from the *Vinca rosea* plant (periwinkle). They bind strongly to tubulin, a class of proteins that form the mitotic spindle during cell division. They disrupt mitotic spindle formation during mitosis at the metaphase of the cell cycle. Cell death results from an inability to segregate chromosomes. Vinca alkaloids are usually regarded as M-phase specific in the cell cycle.

- Paclitaxel is a naturally occurring chemical that is obtained from the yew tree (genus *Taxus*). It binds specifically and reversibly to tubulin and stabilizes microtubules in the polymerized form. Stabilization of microtubules disrupts mitosis and kills cells.

- Docetaxel is a semisynthetic anticancer drug that belongs to the taxoid family. It is a mitotic spindle poison that increases the rate of microtubule assembly and inhibits the depolymerization of microtubules.

- Etoposide is a semisynthetic derivative of podophyllotoxin that is produced in the roots of the American mandrake, or May apple. Its mechanism of action is poorly understood. However, it produces a single-strand breakage of DNA. Etoposide is most lethal to cells in the S and G_2 phases of the cell cycle.

Hormones and Drugs that Affect Hormones

Estrogens, progestins, androgens, and corticosteroids are used in the treatment of various cancers.

- Estrogens are employed in the treatment of prostatic cancer and in the management of five-year postmenopausal breast tumors.
- Androgens are sometimes given to premenopausal patients with mammary cancer.
- Progestins are used on occasion to treat kidney and endometrial carcinomas.
- Corticosteroids, particularly prednisone, are administered in high doses to patients with lymphomas and some other cancers.

The rationale behind the use of these drugs is the belief that some cancers are hormone dependent. For example, if a prostatic cancer is androgen dependent, treatment with estrogens, together with castration, may be reasonable. The converse is also true. If breast cancer in premenopausal patients is estrogen dependent, the use of androgens may make sense. Corticosteroids induce a regression of lymphoid tissue by causing a breakdown of existing lymphocytes and inhibiting the production of new lymphocytes.

- Tamoxifen competitively blocks estrogen receptors. Certain forms of cancer, notably breast cancer in premenopausal women, often depend on endogenous estrogens for growth. When given in high doses, tamoxifen prevents endogenous estrogens from stimulating their receptors and significantly reduces cancer growth.
- Flutamide inhibits androgen uptake and/or nuclear binding of androgen in target tissues. Flutamide is used in combination with luteinizing hormone–releasing hormone (LHRH) agonist analogues (such as leuprolide acetate) for the treatment of metastatic prostatic carcinoma.
- Leuprolide and buserelin are synthetic derivatives of gonadotropin-releasing hormone (GnRH/LHRH). Chronic exposure of the pituitary to these agents abolishes gonadotropin release and results in markedly decreased estrogen and testosterone produced by the gonads. These drugs are used for palliative treatment of patients with hormone-dependent advanced carcinoma of the prostate. They are also useful in breast cancer.
- Goserelin acetate is also a synthetic analogue of GnRH. Administered chronically, goserelin inhibits gonadotropin production, resulting in gonadal and accessory sex organ regression. Goserelin is approved for the palliative treatment of patients with hormone-dependent advanced carcinoma of the prostate.

Miscellaneous Antineoplastics

Asparaginase is an enzyme extracted from cultures of *Escherichia coli*. It converts asparagine to aspartic acid. Certain cancers are unable to make asparagine and are dependent on the blood to bring them adequate amounts of asparagine. In the absence of asparagine, because of its hydrolysis to aspartic acid by asparaginase, the cells cannot proliferate. Asparaginase is not toxic to normal cells, which have the ability to synthesize asparagine.

Procarbazine is converted to an active metabolite in the liver of patients. Following activation, it can cause chromosomal damage and suppress DNA, RNA, and protein synthesis.

ADVERSE EFFECTS OF ANTINEOPLASTIC DRUGS

Antineoplastic drugs are cellular poisons that kill both malignant and normal cells. As previously stated, the selective toxicity seen with antibiotics—in which the drug preferentially attacks the microbe, leaving the host largely unaffected—is not seen with antineoplastics. For example, a drug that blocks DNA or RNA synthesis and/or function will damage both normal and malignant cells. This is particularly true for cell-cycle independent drugs. Cell-cycle dependent drugs will also damage both normal and neoplastic tissue, but these agents show a selectivity for tissues with the highest percentage of cells "in cycle." This means that they can rapidly kill both cancer cells and normal cells with a rapid turnover (eg, bone marrow, GI tract, hair). They also damage the immune system, resulting in a fall in the production of both T and B lymphocytes.

Particular Systems At Risk

The hematopoietic system is particularly at risk when antineoplastic drugs are administered. Patients often show pancytopenia as the production of red cells, white cells, and platelets decreases. The decrease in platelets predisposes patients to hemorrhage. A decrease in neutrophils, together with the fall in B and T lymphocytes, places patients at risk of infections.

The mucosal cells of hollow organs normally have a rapid rate of turnover. By inhibiting cell duplication, antineoplastics damage the GI and genitourinary (GU) tracts, leading to ulceration and bleeding.

Hair and **nails** are damaged by antineoplastics and alopecia and baldness are common adverse effects.

Antineoplastics increase tissue breakdown, raising both the purine load and the production of uric acid, possibly leading to kidney damage.

Some antineoplastics can produce significant nerve damage. Vinca alkaloids do this by interfering with microtubular structures important to nerve function.

Anticancer drugs often produce **nausea** and **vomiting**. These effects are particularly pronounced with cisplatin.

Doxorubicin and daunomycin can cause **cardiac arrhythmias** and, eventually, **heart failure**.

Procarbazine is metabolized to a monoamine oxidase inhibitor and can produce the **CNS effects** characteristic of these drugs (see Chapter 21). Patients should be warned to refrain from eating or drinking foods containing tyramine (eg, cheese, red wine).

Index

Note: Page numbers followed by (t) indicate tables; those followed by (f) indicate figures.

A

Abacavir, 278–281, 278t
Acarbose, 150
ACE inhibitors. *See* Angiotensin-converting enzyme (ACE) inhibitors
Acebutolol, 57–59, 58t, 79–80t, 85, 93–94
Acetaminophen, 218–220, 219f
Acetohexamide, 147–148
Acetylcholine
 actions of, 21
 inactivation of, 22, 23f
 role in parkinsonism, 203–205, 205f
 synthesis of, 22, 23f
Acetylsalicylic acid (ASA)
 actions of, 131, 131f, 215–216, 215f, 221–222
 adverse effects of, 216–218

metabolism of, 217f
pharmacokinetics, 216
uses of, 131, 216
Acids, 2
Acyclovir, 285
Adenosine, 89
Adrenal corticosteroid(s). *See* Glucocorticoid(s); Mineralocorticoids; Sex hormones
Adrenal insufficiency, 156
Adrenaline. *See* Epinephrine
Adrenergic drugs. *See also* Epinephrine; Norepinephrine
 classifications of, 39f
 directly acting, 37, 38f
 indirectly acting, 49
 structures of, 39f
Adrenergic receptor blockers, 51, 55–61
Adrenergic receptor(s), 25–26, 38f
Agonist(s), 13–15, 15f
AIDS. *See* HIV/AIDS
Akathisia, from antipsychotics, 172t
Albuterol/salbutamol, 45–46
Aldosterone

effect on reabsorption, 113
synthesis and secretion of, 157
Alfentanil, 211–214
Alkylating agents, 293–294, 294t
Allopurinol, 227
Alpha and beta blocker(s), 60–61, 103
Alpha blockers
 actions of, 51, 52f, 55–56
 combined with other antihypertensive drugs, 105–106t
 for hypertension, 103
 uses of, 55–56
Alpha$_1$ postsynaptic receptors, 25, 38f
Alpha$_2$ presynaptic receptors, 26, 38f
Alpha-methyldopa, 54, 54f, 104
Alpha-methyltryosine, 51, 53
Alprazolam, 184–189
Alteplase, 135
Amantadine, 209, 285–286
Amdinocillin, 234f, 243
Amdinocillin pivoxal, 243